The Vital Glutes

Connecting the Gait Cycle to Pain and Dysfunction

John Gibbons

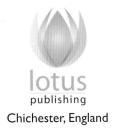

lotus
publishing

Chichester, England

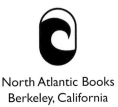

North Atlantic Books
Berkeley, California

First published in 2014 by
Lotus Publishing
Apple Tree Cottage, Inlands Road, Nutbourne, Chichester, PO18 8RJ and
North Atlantic Books
P.O. Box 12327
Berkeley, California 94712

Drawings Amanda Williams
Photographs Ian Taylor
Text Design Wendy Craig
Cover Design Paula Morrison
Printed and Bound in Malaysia by Tien Wah Press

MEDICAL DISCLAIMER: The following information is intended for general information purposes only. Individuals should always see their health care provider before administering any suggestions made in this book. Any application of the material set forth in the following pages is at the reader's discretion and is his or her sole responsibility.

The Vital Glutes: Connecting the Gait Cycle to Pain and Dysfunction is sponsored by the Society for the Study of Native Arts and Sciences, a nonprofit educational corporation whose goals are to develop an educational and crosscultural perspective linking various scientific, social, and artistic fields; to nurture a holistic view of arts, sciences, humanities, and healing; and to publish and distribute literature on the relationship of mind, body, and nature.

British Library Cataloguing-in-Publication Data
A CIP record for this book is available from the British Library
ISBN 978 1 905367 49 8 (Lotus Publishing)
ISBN 978 1 58394 847 7 (North Atlantic Books)

Library of Congress Cataloguing-in-Publication Data
Gibbons, John, 1968- author.
  The vital glutes : connecting the gait cycle to pain and dysfunction / John Gibbons.
    p. ; cm.
  Summary: "Health & Fitness; Alternative Therapies; Pain Management; Exercise"—Provided by publisher.
  ISBN 978-1-58394-847-7 (paperback) — ISBN 978-1-58394-848-4 (ebook)
  I. Society for the Study of Native Arts and Sciences, sponsoring body. II. Title.
  [DNLM: 1. Gait—physiology. 2. Musculoskeletal Pain—etiology. 3. Buttocks—pathology. 4. Musculoskeletal Physiological Phenomena. 5. Physical Therapy Modalities. 6. Range of Motion, Articular. WE 141]
  QP321
  612.7'4--dc23
                                2014014077

Contents

*I dedicate this book to my father, John Andrew Gibbons,
who I wish was here to see what I have achieved,
and to my mother, Margaret Gibbons,
whom I love dearly.*

Preface

The success of my first book, *Muscle Energy Techniques: A Practical Guide for Physical Therapists*, inspired me to continue with the dream of writing, and I wanted to write specifically about what I feel is one of the most neglected areas in physical therapy—the "glutes." The last chapter of my previous book looked at the functions of the gluteus maximus (Gmax) and the gluteus medius (Gmed) and how they affected the gait pattern and subsequently caused pain and dysfunction elsewhere in the body. I also briefly discussed the firing patterns of the specific movements of hip extension and hip abduction. However, I would now like to elaborate upon this fascinating area and hopefully in this book I will do just that. I also want my readers to be able to demonstrate, and explain among their patients and colleagues in discussion groups, that if a weakness or misfiring occurs within these particular firing sequences, a dysfunctional pattern can develop through the body's natural compensatory mechanisms.

In this book I want to take the reader on a journey, just as I did in my first book. The feedback I have received in response to that book has been overwhelming; people have said that the way I have explained things has guided them on their journey through the topic. I consider my books (and also my teaching and articles) to be a bit like jigsaw puzzles: when you first open the box/cover, you have many pieces to try to fit together to form a picture. After reading one chapter you will store some information in your brain, but the "picture" will be somewhat blurred. As you continue reading successive chapters, however, I truly hope a sharper picture will begin to form. Once the book has been read from cover to cover, you should have a clear picture; it might not be crystal clear, but hopefully will be adequate for you to utilize and adapt to your own clinical setting.

I will expand on the theory of muscle weakness and misfiring in order to discuss and demonstrate how and why these issues cause pain and dysfunction in so many patients and athletes. I have also added complementary treatment protocols that will help a physical therapist deal with the causes of the weakness and misfiring, rather than simply treating the symptoms. Once all this has been understood and the causes have been dealt with, I then want the physical therapist to be able to competently advise the athlete/patient on the best forms of gluteal control by the use of specific exercises.

I have now reached a stage where, in almost each and every one of the physical therapy courses I teach (even in the case of the "Shoulder Joint Master Class"), I am constantly being asked about the glutes and how they cause pain in a specific area. I always discuss verbally how this phenomenon can happen and then go on to demonstrate practically the causes and effects; however, I have never been able to say, "Read such-and-such a book and you will find the answer." My aim in writing now is to meet the need for a book which does give such answers. I wanted to produce a text that over time will help many thousands of physical therapists, whether they are students in this area or have been practicing physical therapists for many years. I believe that this book can serve as a core text for anyone in the field of physical therapy who wants a better understanding of how maximizing the glutes to achieve optimum functionality will help reduce a patient's pain and dysfunction in almost every part of the body!

Many years ago I wrote an article called "Putting maximus back into the gluteus." I have written numerous articles over the years but I consider this particular one to be my most important: it has been read by lots of physical therapists throughout the world, and I have had many comments and numerous emails from therapists (and patients too) about the content. I enjoyed producing the article so much so that I decided to write a book on the subject of the glutes, and hence this practical guide for physical therapists on maximizing the glutes.

A revised version of that article forms the first chapter of this book, and I would like to think that reading it will inspire you and whet your appetite to keep on reading. Hopefully you will continue on the journey with me through the remainder of the book, which will go into great depth as to why glute-related pain and dysfunction can present itself in your athletes or patients.

A three-week holiday in Turkey was a good time for me to put pen to paper. Much as I like the sun, it is not a great idea for me to spend all my time in the sunshine, as I have had some skin cancer issues in the past (in fact my father died of skin cancer); so this was a great opportunity to do some writing. While I was sitting there one morning with a coffee, typing on my laptop, my son Thomas came up to me and asked me what I was doing. He knew that I had written a book the previous year, and I had mentioned to him that I was thinking of writing another one just on the glutes, but I am not sure if he understood me at the time. I said I was starting to write the book that I had mentioned to him a while back, but trying to explain to a 12-year-old about the Gmax and Gmed was going to be a bit heavy, so I told him that I was writing a book about the "bum" muscles. He said, "Dad, you are writing a whole book just about the bum muscles?" I replied "Yes," to which my son then responded, "But the bum is just big and a bit squidgy"!

As we now begin our journey, I hope to inspire you to continue reading all the chapters so that you will gain a better understanding of the role of the glutes. Once you have finished the book, you will then realize that there is more to the bum than being "just big and a bit squidgy."

Acknowledgments

My thanks to Jon Hutchings of Lotus Publishing for allowing me the opportunity to continue with my passion for writing—I hope that this book will be as successful as my previous book on muscle energy techniques.

I also want to thank the models and Jack Meeks from Oxford University Sport, as well as Ian Taylor, who spent so much time taking and editing the photographs for this book.

I would like to personally thank someone who guided me through my osteopathy training—a musculoskeletal physiotherapist by the name of Gordon Bosworth. I consider him to be one of the best, if not *the* best, physical therapists I have ever met. He was and still is an inspiration to me in becoming the person I am today.

I have to mention my son, Thomas Rhys Gibbons, as he means the world to me. He was 12 years old at the time of writing this book and without him I would not have had the motivation or dedication to achieve what I have accomplished in my life so far. I have many dreams and aspirations in my life and one of them is to be a success in any avenue or goal that I pursue. That is one of the reasons I do what I do in my life, as I want to show my son that when you set your heart on achieving something that you might initially consider to be potentially unachievable, then with continued perseverance you will notice that things start to change in your life, and your dream eventually becomes a reality.

I would like to think that, in times to come, my son will look back at the books I have written, and which have been personally dedicated to him, and feel that since his dad has accomplished some things in his life even though it took him a while to get started, he will easily be able to do the same. You just need a goal in your life, and to add some passion to the equation, and then anything—and I mean anything—can be achieved. I am hoping that my success and determination will inspire and motivate him to do well in his own life.

Thanks too to my sister, Amanda Williams, and her family. I truly hope for all the success that you, and your gorgeous children, James and Victoria (who I have seen growing up over the years and are aspiring to be amazing teenagers), deserve—and long may it last!

And, finally, a big thank you to my fiancée, Denise Thomas, who has stuck with me over the years and regularly puts up with my grumpy tantrum days. You have unfailingly encouraged and guided me over the last few years, and also allowed me the freedom to pursue my dreams. Without you this book would not have been possible.

John Gibbons

List of Abbreviations

ACJ	acromioclavicular joint
AHC	anterior horn cell
AROM	active range of motion
ASIS	anterior superior iliac spine
ATFL	anterior talofibular ligament
CFL	calcaneofibular ligament
CKC	closed kinetic chain
COG	center of gravity
DDD	degenerative disc disease
EMG	electromyography
GTO	Golgi tendon organ
ILA	inferior lateral angle
ITB	iliotibial band
ITBFS	iliotibial band friction syndrome
LLD	leg length discrepancy
MCL	medial collateral ligament
MET	muscle energy technique
MRI	magnetic resonance imaging
MVIC	maximal voluntary isometric contraction
OA	osteoarthritis
OKC	open kinetic chain
PD	pelvic drop
PFPS	patellofemoral pain syndrome
PHC	posterior horn cell
PIR	post-isometric relaxation
PLS	posterior longitudinal sling
PRE	progressive resistance exercise
PROM	passive range of motion
PSIS	posterior superior iliac spine
QL	quadratus lumborum
RI	reciprocal inhibition
ROM	range of motion
SCJ	sternoclavicular joint
SCM	sternocleidomastoid
SIJ	sacroiliac joint
STJ	subtalar joint
TFL	tensor fasciae latae
TLF	thoracolumbar fascia
TMJ	temporomandibular joint
TVA	transversus abdominis
VM	vastus medialis
VMO	vastus medialis oblique
WP	wall press
WS	wall squat

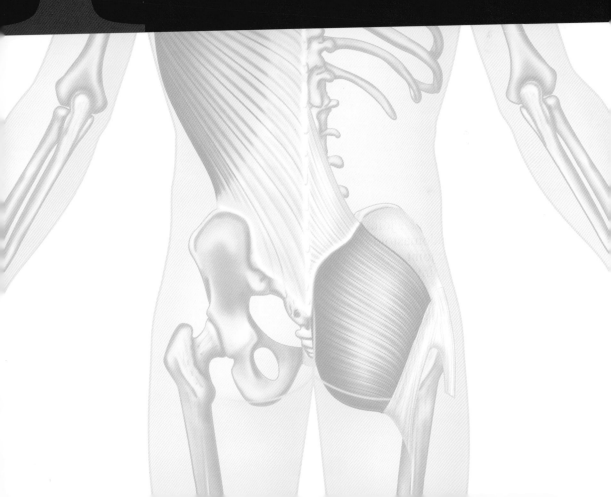

1 Putting the Maximus Back into Gluteus Maximus

Physical therapists are what I call *detectives*: they possess some clues (patient's history and symptoms), but they then have to take the patient through an elimination process (via a physical assessment) to hopefully find out and identify the actual underlying cause of the symptoms. The purpose of this chapter is to briefly explain about a patient who presented with pain in the left shoulder area, and to demonstrate that the possible cause of the problem can originate in an area that one might not consider in view of the patient's presenting symptoms.

This chapter hopefully demonstrates what Dr. Ida Rolf states—"Where you think the pain is, the problem is not." I want to illustrate this statement from Dr. Rolf with a case study taken from my own physical therapy clinic at the University of Oxford. As I become more experienced, not only in lecturing physical therapy courses but also as a practicing sports osteopath in my own clinic, I am convinced that many issues which patients and athletes present with are purely symptoms rather than actual causes. This was one of the main driving forces that inspired me to write the article "Putting maximus back into the gluteus" (Gibbons 2009), on which this chapter is based, and that has naturally led to the writing of a whole book on the subject.

The case study below is just a small snippet of the information that I provide in this book. The information contained within the study is taken from a real case study patient who came to my clinic for a consultation.

Case Study

The patient in question was a woman of 34 and a physical trainer for the Royal Air Force. She presented to the clinic with pain near the superior aspect of her left scapula (figure 1.1). The pain would come on four miles into a run, forcing her to stop because it was so intense. The discomfort would then subside, but quickly return if she attempted to start running again. Running was the only activity that caused the pain. Her complaint had been ongoing for eight months, had worsened over the past three, and was starting to affect her work. There was no previous history or related trauma to trigger the complaint.

After seeing different practitioners, who all focused their treatment on the upper trapezius, she visited an osteopath who treated her cervical spine and rib area. The treatments she had received were biased toward the application of soft tissue techniques to the affected area, namely the trapezius, levator scapulae, sternocleidomastoid (SCM), scalenes, and so on. The osteopath had also used manipulative techniques on the facet joints of her cervical spine—C4/5 and C5/6. Muscle energy techniques and trigger point releases were used in a localized area, which offered relief at the time but made no difference when she attempted to run more than four miles. She had not undergone any scans (e.g. MRI or x-ray).

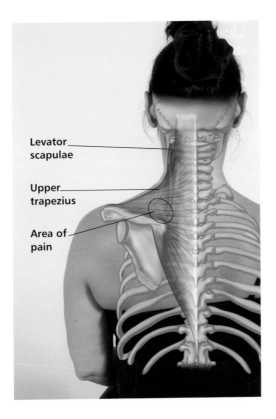

Figure 1.1: Diagram of painful area—left superior scapula.

Assessment

During a consultation (subjective history) the physical therapist will ask specific questions relating to the patient's presenting pain so that a picture can be formed in their mind. This is a normal process in order for the physical therapist to come up with a hypothesis; this type of initial diagnosis will then help the therapist decide on what tissue(s) might be responsible for causing the client's presenting pain/ symptoms. For the patient in question, the potential tissues responsible for the pain to her superior scapula are:

- Upper trapezius

- Levator scapulae

- Scalenes

- Thoracic rib

- Cervical rib (extra rib forming from the transverse process of C7)

Once a subjective history has been conducted, the physical therapist then proceeds to an objective assessment: this is where the therapist uses specialized techniques to assess the musculoskeletal system to come up with a thorough diagnosis. One of the specific techniques employed by the therapist can be simple range of motion (ROM) tests that are initially performed by the patient; these are known as *active range of motion (AROM)* tests. This assessment is generally followed by a series of *passive range of motion (PROM)* tests; these tests are normally performed on the patient by the therapist, and are commonly used to check the integrity of the affected joint. Resisted testing comes next: this type of specific movement tests the power and involvement of the contractile tissues, i.e. muscles and tendons. The physical therapist also uses palpatory awareness through their fingertips to decide on the condition of the affected tissues, and will generally include special tests to complement the diagnosis.

The potential causes of my patient's presenting pain are:

- Referral pain from cervical facet C4/5 or C5/6

- Protective spasm/strain of upper trapezius or levator scapulae

- Dysfunction of the glenohumeral joint or even the acromioclavicular joint (ACJ) or sternoclavicular joint (SCJ)

- Intervertebral disc bulge of C4/5 or C5/6

- Elevated first rib

- Cervical rib (extra rib from the transverse process of C7)

- Relative shortness/tightness of the scalenes

- Positional—due to upper crossed syndrome related to a forward head posture and rounded shoulders caused by tight pectorals and SCM, and possibly weak rhomboids and serratus anterior

- Upper lobe of left lung, referring to the trapezius

- Diaphragm—this is innervated by the phrenic nerve, which originates from the level of C3–5 from the cervical spine; the dermatome from C3–5 can cause a referred pattern of pain that can radiate to the area of the shoulder (*dermatome* is an area of skin that is supplied from a single nerve root)

As you can see, there are many possible causes of the patient's presenting pain. This list is not exhaustive and highlights just some of the many avenues to consider when confronted with a common complaint of "shoulder/trapezius pain."

Taking a Holistic Approach

Let's now assess the case study patient globally rather than locally, remembering that the pain only comes on after running four miles.

When I see a new patient for the first time, no matter what the presenting pain is, I normally assess the pelvis for position and movement, as I consider this area of the body in particular to be the "foundation" for everything that connects to it. I often find in clinic that when I correct a dysfunctional pelvis, my client's presenting symptoms tend to settle down. However, when I assessed this particular patient, I found her pelvis was level and moving correctly. I then went on to test the firing patterns of the gluteus maximus (referred to as the *Gmax* for the remainder of this book), which I often do with patients and athletes who participate in regular sporting activities. However, I only test the firing pattern sequence once I feel that the pelvis is in its correct position; the logic here is that you often get a positive result of the muscle misfiring when the pelvis is slightly out of position.

With the patient in question, I found a bilateral weakness/misfiring of the Gmax, but the firing on the right side seemed a bit slower. As I had not found any dysfunction in the pelvis, I pursued this line of approach a little further.

Before we continue I would like to pose a few questions for you to think about:

- How does a weakness of the Gmax on the right side cause pain in the left trapezius?

- Is there a link between the Gmax and the trapezius, and if so, how is this possible?

- What can be done to correct the issue?

- What has happened to cause it in the first place?

To answer these questions, we need to look at the functional anatomy of the Gmax, and the relationship of the Gmax to other anatomical structures, as detailed in later chapters.

Gmax Function

The Gmax operates mainly as a powerful hip extensor and a lateral rotator, but it also plays a part in stabilizing the sacroiliac joint (SIJ) by helping it to "force close" while going through the gait cycle.

Some of the Gmax muscular fibers attach to the sacrotuberous ligament, which runs from the sacrum to the ischial tuberosity (see figure 2.4). This ligament has been termed the *key ligament* in helping to stabilize the SIJ. To gain a better understanding of this action, we first need to consider two concepts—"form closure" and "force closure"—which are both associated with stability of the SIJ (see figure 1.2).

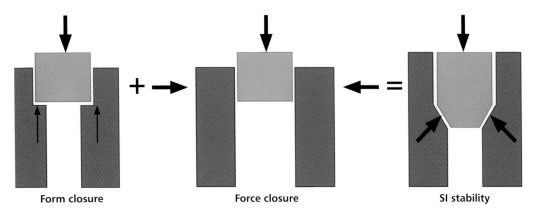

Form closure   **Force closure**   **SI stability**

Figure 1.2: Form closure and force closure.

The shape of the sacrum—along with its ridges and grooves, and the fact that it is wedged between the ilia—helps to bring natural stability to the SIJ. This is known as *form closure*. If the articular surfaces of the sacrum and the ilia fitted together with perfect form closure, mobility would be practically nonexistent. However, form closure of the SIJ is not perfect and movement is possible, which means stabilization during loading is required. This is achieved by increasing compression across the joint at the moment of loading; the surrounding ligaments, muscles, and fascia are responsible for this. The mechanism of compression of the SIJ by these additional forces is called *force closure*.

When the body is working efficiently, the forces between the innominates and the sacrum are adequately controlled, and loads can be transferred between the trunk, pelvis, and legs. So how do we link this to the patient's complaint? In one of my previous articles (Gibbons 2008), about training the Oxford rowing team, I wrote about the posterior oblique "sling." This structure directly links the right Gmax to the left latissimus dorsi via the thoracolumbar fascia (figure 1.3). The latissimus dorsi has its insertion on the inner part of the humerus, and one of the functions of this muscle is to keep the scapula against the thoracic cage and aid in depression of the scapula.

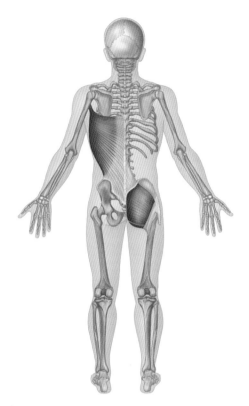

Figure 1.3: Posterior oblique sling.

Piecing It All Together

So what do we know? We know that the right side of the patient's Gmax is slightly slower in terms of its firing pattern and that this muscle plays a role in the force closure process of the SIJ. This tells us that if the Gmax cannot perform this function of stabilizing the SIJ, then something else will assist in stabilizing the joint. The left latissimus dorsi is the synergist that helps stabilize the right Gmax and, more importantly, the SIJ. As the patient participates in running, every time her right leg contacts the ground and goes through the gait cycle, the left latissimus dorsi is over-contracting. This causes the left scapula to depress, and the muscles that resist the downward depressive pull will be the upper trapezius and the levator scapulae. Subsequently, these muscles start to fatigue; for the patient in question, this occurs at approximately four miles, at which point she feels pain in her left superior scapula.

Treatment

You might think the easy way to treat the weakness in the Gmax is to simply prescribe strength-based exercises. However, in practice this is not always the correct solution, as sometimes the tighter antagonistic muscle is responsible for the apparent weakness. The muscle in this case is the iliopsoas (hip flexor), and shortening of this can result in a weakness inhibition of the Gmax. My answer to this puzzle was to stretch the patient's right iliopsoas muscle to see if it promoted the firing activation of the Gmax, while at the same time introducing strength exercises for the Gmax. All this will be explained in more detail in chapter 8 and chapter 12.

Prognosis and Conclusion

I advised the patient to abstain from running and to get her partner to assist in lengthening the iliopsoas, rectus femoris, and adductors twice a day. Strength exercises were also advised twice daily until the follow-on treatment (these exercises are discussed in later chapters). I reassessed her 10 days later and found normal firing of the Gmax on the hip extension firing pattern test, and a reduction in the tightness of the associated iliopsoas, rectus femoris, and adductors. Because of these positive results, I advised her to run as far as felt comfortable. I was not sure if my treatment was going to correct the problem, but she reported that she had no pain during or after a six-mile run. The patient is still pain free and continues to regularly use the Gmax strengthening exercises and the lengthening techniques for the tight muscles.

This case study demonstrates that very often the underlying cause of a condition or problem may not be local to where the symptoms/pain presents, which means that all avenues need to be fully considered. I hope that the information from this study has intrigued you enough to continue reading, as the information presented is just a taster of what is to come in the following chapters. Remember, this book is what I call a *jigsaw puzzle journey*—if you stick with it, the picture will eventually become a lot clearer.

Muscle Imbalance and the Myofascial Slings

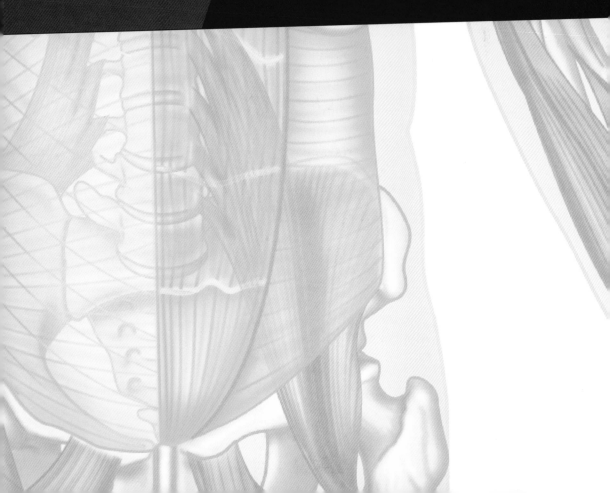

This chapter will cover muscle imbalance, which I feel is very relevant to the potential problems that can contribute to dysfunctional glutes. Even though I do not refer to the individual muscles of the glutes very often, it is still necessary to understand the function of the various types of muscle and, more importantly, how they can influence the position of the body. If we experience pain we can safely assume that we most likely have dysfunction somewhere in our body; if there is dysfunction we can say that we have an imbalance, and if we have an imbalance then I can guarantee that the glutes will be involved somewhere in this dysfunctional process.

People are commonly considered to be "creatures of habit": we like to repeat things on a regular basis so that they become "normal." Let's take, for example, the iliopsoas muscle; I personally believe that this muscle is constantly in a "forced shortened" position for most of the time, because after getting up in the morning we naturally sit down at the kitchen table to have breakfast, get into our cars, and drive to work. On arrival at work most of us will sit at a desk for much of the day. We even sit down when we have lunch or a break. At the end of the working day we get back in the car and drive home, and then sit down for an evening meal, before relaxing and sitting either in an armchair or on the sofa to watch TV. When we eventually make it to bed, many of us find that the only comfortable sleeping position is on our side in a sort of fetal position, further exacerbating the problem. When we wake up, the whole process is repeated.

I am sure that by now it has become obvious to you that the iliopsoas muscle is naturally being forced into a shortened position for most of the day as a result of our repetitive habits and lifestyles. You will read in later chapters that because this muscle is being held in this unnatural shortened position, it will eventually become a tight structure. A tightness of the iliopsoas can therefore be one of the pieces in the "jigsaw puzzle" and can be a vital clue to a patient's presenting symptoms. The iliopsoas might be the "key" to unlocking the problem because if left in a shortened position, the length of its antagonist muscle—in this case the glutes—will potentially be altered. If this muscle group is continually held in a lengthened position for an extended period of time then subsequent weakening ensues.

Posture

Definition: *Posture* is the attitude or position of the body (Thomas 1997).

According to Martin (2002), posture should fulfill three functions:

- Maintaining the alignment of the body's segments in any position: supine, prone, sitting, all fours, and standing

- Anticipating change to allow engagement in voluntary, goal-directed movements, such as reaching and stepping

- Reacting to unexpected perturbations or disturbances in balance

From the above, it can be seen that posture is an active as well as a purely static state and that it is synonymous with balance. Optimal posture must be maintained at all times, not only when holding static positions (e.g. sitting and standing) but also during movement.

If optimal posture and postural control are to be encouraged during exercise performance, the principles of good static posture must be fully appreciated. Once these are understood, poor posture can be identified and corrective strategies adopted.

- *Good posture* is the state of muscular and skeletal balance that protects the supporting structures of the body against injury or progressive deformity, irrespective of the attitude (e.g. erect, lying, squatting, or stooping) in which these structures are working or resting.

- *Poor posture* is a faulty relationship of the various parts of the body, which produces increased strain on the supporting structures and in which there is less efficient balance of the body over its base of support.

The neuromuscular system, as we know, is made up of *slow-twitch* and *fast-twitch* muscle fibers, each having a different role in the body's function. Slow-twitch fibers (Type I) are for sustained low-level activity, such as maintaining correct posture, whereas fast-twitch fibers (Type II) are for powerful, gross movements. Muscles can also be broken down into two further categories—*tonic* (or *postural*) and *phasic*.

Tonic (Postural) and Phasic Muscles

Janda (1987) identified two groups of muscles on the basis of their evolution and development. Functionally, muscles can be classified as *tonic* or *phasic*. The tonic system consists of the flexors, which develop later on to become the dominant structure. Umphred (2001) identified that the tonic muscles are involved in repetitive or rhythmic activity and are activated in flexor synergies, whereas the phasic system consists of the extensors and emerges shortly after birth. The phasic muscles work eccentrically against the force of gravity and are involved in extensor synergies. The division of muscles into predominantly phasic and predominantly postural is given in table 2.1, overleaf.

Predominantly postural muscles	Predominantly phasic muscles
Shoulder girdle	
Pectoralis major/minor	Rhomboids
Levator scapulae	Lower trapezius
Upper trapezius	Mid trapezius
Biceps brachii	Seratus anterior
Neck extensors: Scalenes / Cervical erectors / Sternocleidomastoid	Triceps brachii
	Neck flexors: Supra- and infrahyoid / Longus colli
Lower arm	
Wrist flexors	Wrist extensors
Trunk	
Lumbar and cervical erectors	Thoracic erectors
Quadratus lumborum	Abdominals
Pelvis	
Biceps femoris / Semitendinosus / Semimembranosus	Vastus medialis
Iliopsoas	Vastus lateralis
ITB	Gluteus maximus
Rectus femoris	Gluteus minimus and medius
Adductors	
Piriformis / Tensor fasciae latae	
Lower leg	
Gastrocnemius / Soleus	Tibialis anterior / Peroneals

Table 2.1: Phasic and postural muscles of the body.

Previous authors have suggested that muscles which have a stabilizing function (postural) have a natural tendency to shorten when stressed, and that other muscles which play a more active/moving role (phasic) have a tendency to lengthen and can subsequently become inhibited (see table 2.2). The muscles which tend to shorten have a primary postural role and are related to the potential inhibition weakness of the glutes, which you will read about later.

There are some exceptions to the rule which states that certain muscles follow the pattern of becoming shortened while others become lengthened—some muscles are capable of modifying their structure. For example, some authors suggest that the scalenes are postural in nature, while others suggest that they are phasic. We know from specific testing, depending on what dysfunction is present within the muscle framework, that the scalenes can be found to be held in a shortened position and tight, but at other times they can be found to be lengthened and weakened.

There is a distinction between postural and phasic muscles; however, many muscles can display characteristics of both and contain a mixture of Type I and Type II fibers. The hamstring muscles, for example, have a postural stabilizing function, yet are polyarticular (cross more than one joint) and are notoriously prone to shortening.

	Postural	**Phasic**
Function	Posture	Movement
Muscle type	Type I	Type II
Fatigue	Late	Early
Reaction	Shortening	Lengthening

Table 2.2: Lengthening and shortening of muscles.

Postural Muscles

Also known as *tonic* muscles, the postural muscles have an antigravity role and are therefore heavily involved in the maintenance of posture. Slow-twitch fibers are more suited to maintaining posture: they are capable of sustained contraction but generally become shortened and subsequently tight.

Postural muscles are slow-twitch dominant because of their resistance to fatigue, and are innervated by a smaller motor neuron. They therefore have a lower excitability threshold, which means the nerve impulse will reach the postural muscle before the phasic muscle. With this sequence of innervation, the postural muscle will inhibit the phasic (antagonist) muscle, thus reducing its contractile potential and activation.

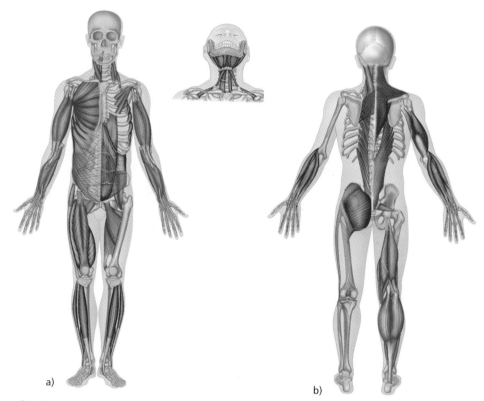

Figure 2.1: Postural and phasic muscles: (a) Anterior view; (b) Posterior view. The blue muscles are predominantly postural, and the red muscles predominantly phasic.

Phasic Muscles

Movement is the main function of phasic muscles. These muscles are often more superficial than postural muscles and tend to be polyarticular. They are composed of predominantly Type II fibers and are under voluntary reflex control.

A shortened, tight muscle often results in inhibition of the associated phasic muscle, whose function becomes weakened as a result. The relationship between a tightness-prone muscle and an associated weakness-prone muscle is one way. As the tightness-prone muscle becomes tighter and subsequently stronger, this causes an inhibition of the weakness-prone muscle, resulting in its lengthening and consequent weakening: think about the previously mentioned relationship between the iliopsoas and the glutes.

Muscle Activity Before and After Stretching

Let's look at some electromyography (EMG) studies of trunk muscle activity before and after stretching hypertonic muscles, in this case the erector spinae. In table 2.3 the hypertonic erector spinae are indicated as being active during trunk flexion. After stretching, these muscles are suppressed both in trunk flexion (which allows greater activation of the rectus abdominis) and in trunk extension.

Muscle	First recording			Second recording		
Rectus abdominis						
Erector spinae						

Table 2.3: EMG recordings of muscle activity. (Source: Hammer 1999)

Effects of Muscle Imbalance

The research results of Janda (1983) indicate that tight or overactive muscles not only hinder the agonist through Sherrington's law of reciprocal inhibition (Sherrington 1907), but also become active in movements that they are not normally associated with. This is the reason why, when trying to correct a musculoskeletal imbalance, you would encourage lengthening of an overactive muscle by using a muscle energy technique (MET), prior to attempting to strengthen a weak elongated muscle.

If muscle imbalances are not addressed, the body will be forced into a compensatory position, which increases the stress placed on the musculoskeletal system, eventually leading to tissue breakdown, irritation, and injury. You are now in a vicious circle of musculoskeletal deterioration as the tonic muscles shorten and the phasic muscles lengthen (table 2.4, overleaf).

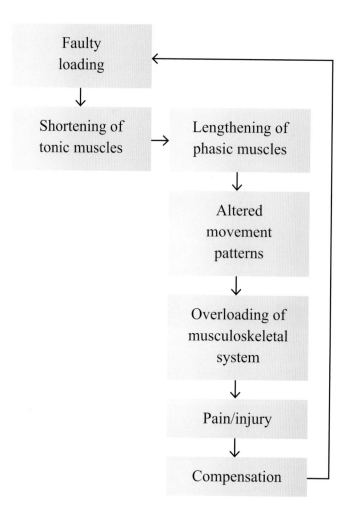

Table 2.4: The vicious circle of musculoskeletal deterioration.

Muscle imbalances are ultimately reflected in posture. As mentioned earlier, postural muscles are innervated by a smaller motor neuron and therefore have a lower excitability threshold. Since the nerve impulse reaches the postural muscle before the phasic muscle, the postural muscle will inhibit the phasic (antagonist) muscle, thus reducing the contractile potential and activation.

When muscles are subject to faulty or repetitive loading, the postural muscles shorten and the phasic muscles weaken, thus altering their length–tension relationship. Consequently, posture is directly affected because the surrounding muscles displace the soft tissues and the skeleton.

Core Muscle Relationships

As the incidence of lower back pain seems to be on the increase, we will need to look at and understand the muscular relationships that affect core and lumbopelvic stability and how METs can be incorporated into the assessment and treatment plan.

The pelvis, or SIJ to be more precise, has two main factors that affect its stability:

- Form closure
- Force closure

Form Closure

Form closure arises from the anatomical alignment of the bones of the innominate and the sacrum, where the sacrum forms a kind of keystone between the wings of the pelvis. The SIJ transfers large loads and its shape is adapted to this task. The articular surfaces are relatively flat and this helps to transfer compression forces and bending movements. However, a relatively flat joint is vulnerable to shear forces. The SIJ is protected from these forces in three ways. First, the sacrum is wedge shaped and thus is stabilized by the innominates. Second, in contrast to other synovial joints, the articular cartilage is not smooth but rather irregular. Third, a frontal dissection through the SIJ reveals cartilage- covered bone extensions protruding into the joint—the so-called "ridges" and "grooves." They seem irregular, but are in fact complementary, and this serves to stabilize the joint when compression is applied.

Force Closure

If the articular surfaces of the sacrum and the innominates fitted together with perfect form closure, mobility would be practically impossible. However, form closure of the SIJ is not perfect and mobility is possible, albeit small, and therefore stabilization during loading is required. This is achieved by increasing compression across the joint at the moment of loading; the anatomical structures responsible for this compression are the ligaments, muscles, and fasciae. The mechanism of compression of the SIJ by these additional forces is called *force closure*. When the SIJ is compressed, friction of the joint increases and consequently reinforces form closure.

Sacroiliac Stability

Several ligaments, muscles, and fascial systems contribute to force closure of the pelvis: collectively these have been called the *osteoarticular-ligamentous system*. Recall that when the body is working efficiently, the shear forces between the innominates and the sacrum are adequately controlled and loads can be transferred between the trunk, pelvis, and legs.

As you will read later on, the Gmax plays a highly significant role in stabilizing the sacroiliac joints, as some of the Gmax fibers merge and attach onto the sacrotuberous ligament as well as onto a connective tissue structure known as the *thoracolumbar fascia (TLF)*. The Gmax connects, via the TLF, to the contralateral latissimus dorsi to form what is known as the *posterior oblique myofascial sling* (see section "The Outer Core Unit: The Integrated Myofascial Sling System" below). Weakness, or possibly a misfiring sequence, of the Gmax will predispose the sacroiliac joint to injury by decreasing the function of this (posterior oblique) myofascial sling. A weakness or misfiring of the Gmax is a potential cause of a compensatory overactivation of the contralateral latissimus dorsi; walking and running (gait cycle) impose high loads on the sacroiliac joint, so this weight-bearing joint will need to be stabilized because of the altered compensatory mechanism.

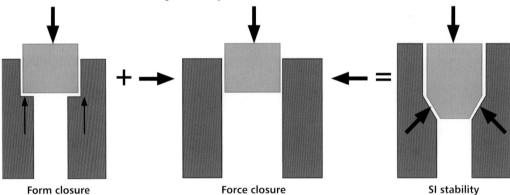

| Form closure | Force closure | SI stability |

Figure 2.2: The relationship between form/force closure and sacroiliac stability.

In which position is the pelvic girdle the most stable? Research has shown that sacral nutation (a nodding type of movement of the sacrum between the innominates) occurs when moving, for example, from a sitting position to standing, and that full nutation occurs during forward or backward bending of the trunk. This motion of sacral nutation tightens the major ligaments (sacrotuberous, sacrospinous, and interosseous) of the posterior pelvis, and this tension increases the compressive force across the SIJ. The increased tension provides the required stability that is needed by the SIJ during the gait cycle as well as when simply rising from a sitting position to standing.

Sacral Nutation and Counternutation

Osar (2012) mentions that *nutation* is the anterior inferior motion of the sacral base, while *counternutation* is the posterior superior motion of the sacral base. Nutation is necessary for the locking of the SIJ during unilateral stance. The inability to nutate the sacrum is a leading cause of unilateral stance instability and one of the causes of the classic Trendelenburg gait. Counternutation, on the other hand, is necessary in order to unlock the SIJ to allow anterior rotation of the innominate and extension of the hip joint. Inability to unlock or counternutate the sacrum leads to compensatory increases in lumbopelvic flexion, which in turn leads to and perpetuates lumbar instability.

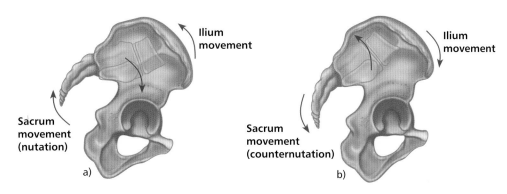

Figure 2.3: (a) Posterior pelvic rotation and sacral nutation;
(b) Anterior pelvic rotation and sacral counternutation.

Force Closure Ligaments

The main ligamentous structures that influence force closure are the sacrotuberous ligament, which connects the sacrum to the ischium (and has been termed the *key ligament*), and the long dorsal sacroiliac ligament, which connects the third and fourth sacral segments to the posterior superior iliac spine (PSIS) (and also known as the *posterior sacroiliac ligament*).

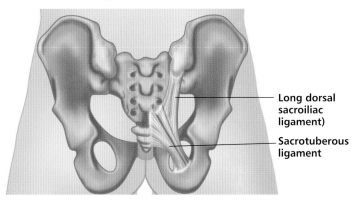

Figure 2.4: Force closure ligaments.

Ligaments can increase articular compression when they are tensed or lengthened by the movement of the bones to which they attach, or when they are tensed by contraction of muscles that insert into the bones. Tension in the sacrotuberous ligament can be increased by posterior rotation of the innominate bone relative to the sacrum, by nutation of the sacrum relative to the innominates, or by contraction of the four muscles—biceps femoris, piriformis, Gmax, and multifidus—that attach to it.

The main ligamentous restraint to counternutation of the sacrum, or anterior rotation of the innominate, is the long dorsal sacroiliac ligament or the posterior sacroiliac ligament. This is a less stable position (compared with the position of nutation) for the pelvis to resist horizontal and/or vertical loading, since the SIJ is under less compression and is not self-locked. The long dorsal ligament is commonly a source of pain and may be palpated just below the level of the PSIS.

By themselves, ligaments cannot maintain a stable pelvis—they rely on several muscle systems to assist them. There are two important groups of muscles that contribute to stability of the lower back and pelvis. Collectively they have been called the *inner unit* (core) and the *outer unit* (myofascial sling systems). The inner unit consists of the transversus abdominis, multifidus, diaphragm, and muscles of the pelvic floor—also collectively known as the *core*, or *local stabilizers*. The outer unit consists of several "slings," or systems of muscles (global stabilizers and mobilisers that are anatomically connected and functionally related).

Force Couple

Definition: A *force couple* is a situation where two forces of equal magnitude, but acting in opposite directions, are applied to an object and pure rotation results (Abernethy et al. 2004).

Any altered positioning of the pelvis caused by potential muscle imbalances will subsequently affect the rest of the kinetic chain. There are several force couples responsible for maintaining proper positioning and alignment of the pelvis. The force couples responsible for controlling the sagittal and frontal planes for the position of the pelvis are shown schematically in figures 2.5 (a–f) and 2.6 (see page 30) respectively.

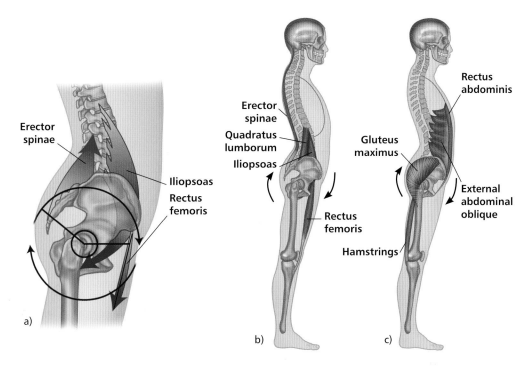

Figure 2.5: (a) Sagittal plane (anterior) pelvic force couple. (b) Anterior tilt: muscles held in a shortened position. (c) Anterior tilt: muscles held in a lengthened position.

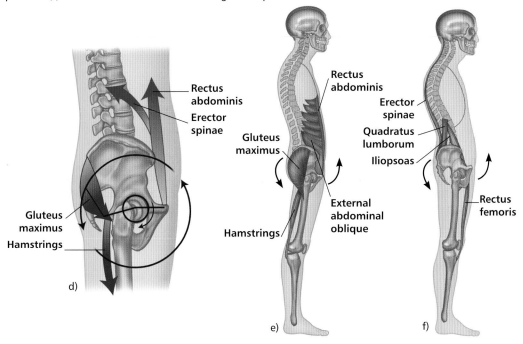

Figure 2.5: (d) Sagittal plane (posterior) pelvic force couple. (e) Posterior tilt: muscles held in a shortened position. (f) Posterior tilt: muscles held in a lengthened position.

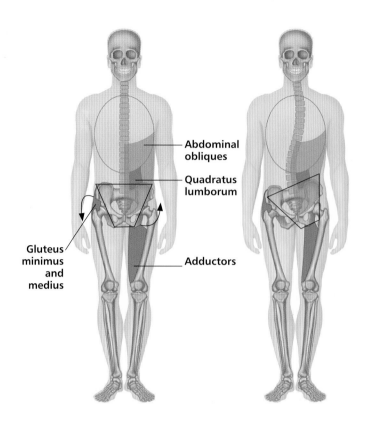

Figure 2.6: Frontal plane (lateral) pelvic force couples.

The Inner Unit: The Core

Definition: *Static stability* is the ability to remain in one position for a long time without losing good structural alignment (Chek 1999).

Static stability is also often referred to as *postural stability*, although this might be somewhat misleading, since as Martin (2002) states: "… posture is more than just maintaining a position of the body such as standing. Posture is active, whether it is in sustaining an existing posture or moving from one posture to another."

The inner unit (figure 2.7) consists of:

- Transversus abdominis
- Multifidus
- Diaphragm
- Muscles of the pelvic floor

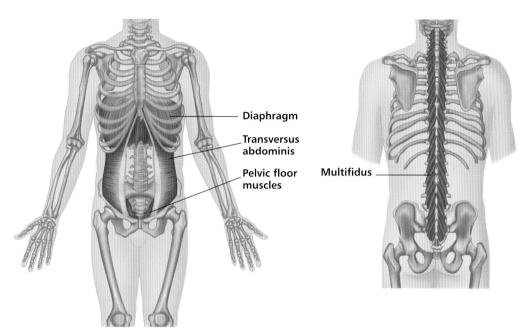

Figure 2.7: The inner unit—the core.

Only the transversus abdominis and multifidus will be covered in this book, as these muscles are specifically related to postural and phasic imbalances and are easily palpated by the physical therapist. Since the diaphragm and muscles of the pelvic floor are difficult to palpate, they will not be discussed here.

Transversus Abdominis

The transversus abdominis (TVA) is the deepest of the abdominal muscles. It originates at the iliac crest, inguinal ligament, lumbar fascia, and associated cartilage of the inferior six ribs, and attaches to the xiphoid process, linea alba, and pubis.

The main action of the TVA is to compress the abdomen via a "drawing-in" of the abdominal wall. This drawing-in is observable as a movement of the umbilicus (belly button) toward the spine. The muscle neither flexes nor extends the spine. Kendall et al. (2010) also state that "this muscle has no action in lateral flexion except that it acts to … stabilize the linea alba, thereby permitting better action by anterolateral trunk muscles [internal and external obliques]."

The TVA appears to be the key muscle of the inner unit. Richardson et al. (1999) found that in people without back pain, the TVA fired 30 milliseconds prior to shoulder movements and 110 milliseconds before leg movements. This corroborates the key role of the TVA in providing the stability necessary to perform movements of the appendicular skeleton. As the TVA contracts during inspiration it pulls the central tendon inferiorly and flattens, thereby increasing the vertical length of the thoracic cavity and compressing the lumbar multifidus.

Multifidus

The multifidus is the most medial of the lumbar back muscles, and its fibers converge near the lumbar spinous processes to an attachment known as the *mammillary process*. The fibers radiate inferiorly, passing to the transverse processes of the vertebrae that lie two, three, four, and five levels below. Those fibers that extend below the level of the last lumbar vertebra (L5) anchor to the ilium and the sacrum. The multifidus is considered to be a series of smaller muscles, which are further divided into superficial and deep components.

The role of the multifidus in producing an extension force is essential to the stability of the lumbar spine, as well as functioning to resist forward flexion of the lumbar spine and the shear forces that are placed upon it. The multifidus muscle also functions to take pressure off the intervertebral discs, so that the body weight is evenly distributed throughout the whole vertebral column. The superficial muscle component acts to keep the vertebral column relatively straight, while the fibers of the deep muscle component contribute to the overall stability of the spine.

Richardson et al. (1999) identified the lumbar multifidus and the TVA as the key stabilizers of the lumbar spine. Both muscles link in with the thoracolumbar fascia to provide what Richardson et al. refer to as "a natural, deep muscle corset to protect the back from injury."

Hydraulic Amplifier

Described by Evan Osar (2012), the hydraulic amplifier effect occurs with the contraction of muscles within their fascial envelopes. All muscles are invested inside fascia and as they contract, push out into the fascia, creating a stiffening around the joint. In the spine, contraction of the lumbar erector spinae and multifidus within the thoracolumbar fascia creates an extension force, assisting extension of the spine. When the lumbosacral multifidus contracts, it broadens posteriorly into the lumbodorsal fascia.

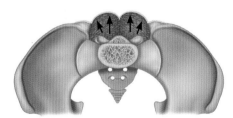

Figure 2.8: As the multifidii contract, it pushes into the thoracolumbar fascia and along with contraction of the transversus abdominis, provides intersegmental stability.

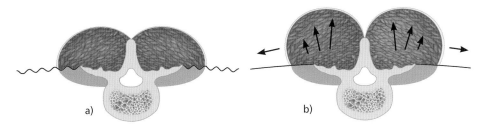

Figure 2.9: a) The relaxed multifidi muscle in transverse section; b) Co-contraction of the transversus abdominis and multifidi creates a stiffening tension on the thoracolumbar fascia thereby providing intersegmental stability.

This effect is aided by contraction of the transversus abdominis, which pulls the thoracolumbar fascia tight around the contracting erector spinae and multifidi, thereby creating a stable column.

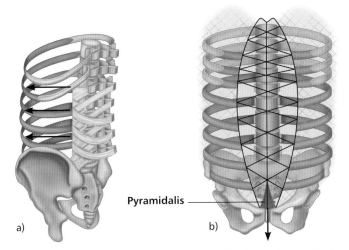

Figure 2.10: a) As the transversus abdominis contracts, it tenses the thoracolumbar fascia, which allows the multifidi and lumbar erector spinae to contract against it and aid spinal elongation and stiffness; b) Contraction of the pyramidalis tenses the linea alba (central tendon), creating a stable base for contraction of the transversus abdominis.

The Outer Core Unit:
The Integrated Myofascial Sling System

The force closure muscles of the outer core unit consist of four myofascial sling systems, known as the *posterior longitudinal*, *lateral*, *anterior oblique*, and *posterior oblique* systems (figures 2.11–2.14). These myofascial slings provide force closure and subsequent stability for the pelvic girdle; failure or even weakness of any of these slings to secure pelvic stability can lead to lumbopelvic pain and dysfunctions. Although the muscles of the outer core unit can be trained individually, effective force closure requires specific co-activation and release for optimal function.

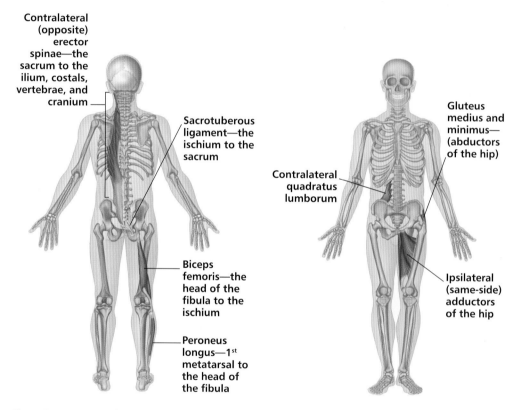

Figure 2.11: Posterior longitudinal system.   Figure 2.12: Lateral system.

The integrated myofascial sling system represents many forces and is composed of several muscles. A muscle may participate in more than one sling, and the slings may overlap and interconnect, depending on the task in hand. There are several slings of myofascial systems in the outer unit, including (but probably not limited to) a *coronal* sling (having medial and lateral components), a *sagittal* sling (having anterior and posterior components), and an *oblique spiral* sling. The hypothesis is that the slings have no beginning or end, but rather connect as necessary to assist in the transference of forces. It is possible that the slings are all part of one interconnected myofascial system, and a sling that is identified during any particular motion could merely be a result of the activation of selective parts of the whole sling (Lee 2004).

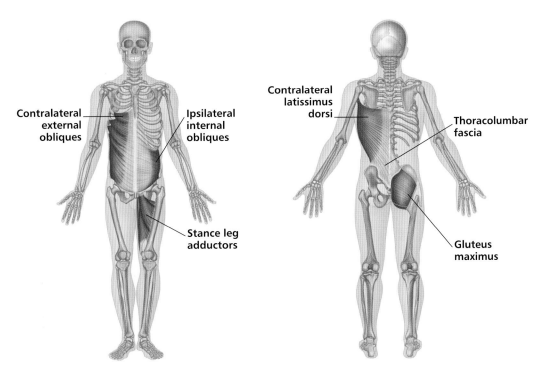

Figure 2.13: Anterior oblique system.   *Figure 2.14: Posterior oblique system.*

The identification and treatment of a specific muscle dysfunction (such as weakness, inappropriate recruitment, or tightness) is important when restoring force closure (second component of stability) and for understanding why parts of a sling may be restricted in motion or lacking in support. Note the following points:

- The four systems of the outer unit are dependent upon the inner unit for the joint stiffness and stability necessary for creating an effective force generation platform.

- Failure of the inner unit to work in the presence of outer unit demand often results in muscle imbalance, joint injury, and poor performance.

- The outer unit cannot be effectively conditioned by the use of modern resistance machines, as the specific training provided by these types of machine generally does not relate to day-to-day functional movements.

- Effective conditioning of the outer unit should include exercises that require integrated function of the inner and outer units, using movement patterns common to any given client's work or sport environment (Chek 1999).

Poor Posture

Poor posture may be a result of many different factors. It may be due to trauma suffered by the body, some form of deformity within the musculoskeletal system, or even faulty loading. Because sitting has become a position that our bodies maintain for long periods of time (possibly 8+ hours), most people in today's society are losing the fight against gravity and altering their center of gravity (COG). With correct posture, the postural muscles are fairly inactive and energy efficient, only responding to disruptions in balance to maintain an upright position. Therefore, as one moves away from ideal alignment, postural muscle tone increases, thus leading to higher energy expenditure.

Sagittal Postural Deviations

Postural deviations can be observed from the sagittal plane, as seen in figures 2.15–2.17. The text highlights which particular muscles are prone to shortening and becoming tight, and those that are prone to lengthening and becoming weak.

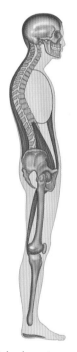

Head:	Forward
Cervical:	Slightly extended
Thoracic:	Lower part straight / upper part flexed
Lumbar:	Flexed (straight)
Pelvis:	Posterior tilt
Hip:	Extended
Knee:	Extended (or flexed)
Ankle:	Slight plantar flexion
Weak and elongated:	Iliopsoas Back extensors (may not be weak)
Short and strong:	Hamstrings

Figure 2.15: Flat-back posture.

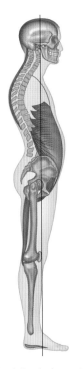

Head:	Forward
Cervical:	Hyperextended
Scapulae:	Abducted
Thoracic:	Hyperkyphosis
Lumbar:	Hyperlordosis
Pelvis:	Anterior tilt
Hip:	Flexed
Knee:	Slightly hyperextended
Ankle:	Slight plantar flexion
Weak and elongated:	Neck flexors
	Upper back
	Hamstrings (may not be weak)
	Obliques
Short and strong:	Neck extensors
	Hip flexors

Figure 2.16: Kyphotic/lordotic posture.

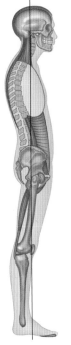

Head:	Forward
Cervical:	Slightly extended
Thoracic:	Flexion (kyphosis)
Lumbar:	Flattened (flexion)
Pelvis:	Posterior tilt
Hip:	Hyperextended and forward
Knee:	Hyperextended
Ankle:	Neutral (pelvis deviation)
Weak and elongated:	Iliopsoas
	Obliques
	Upper back extensors
	Neck flexors
Short and strong:	Hamstrings
	Lower back (not short)
	Upper abdominals

Figure 2.17: Sway-back posture.

Pain Spasm Cycle

Ischemia will be a primary source of pain in the initial stages of poor posture. The blood flow through a muscle is inversely proportional to the level of contraction or activity, reaching almost zero at 50–60% of contraction. Some studies have indicated that the body could not maintain homeostasis with a sustained isometric contraction of over 10%.

The weight of the head is approximately 7% of total body weight (shoulders and arms are around 14%). This means that for a person weighing 176 lb. (80 kg), the head will weigh around 11 to 13 lb. (5 to 6 kg). If the head and shoulders move forward, out of ideal alignment, the activation of the neck extensors will increase dramatically, resulting in restricted blood flow. This prolonged isometric contraction will force the muscles into anaerobic metabolism and increase lactic acid and other irritating metabolite accumulation. If adequate rest is not given, a reflex contraction of the already ischemic muscles may be initiated. This person will have now entered the pain spasm cycle (figure 2.18).

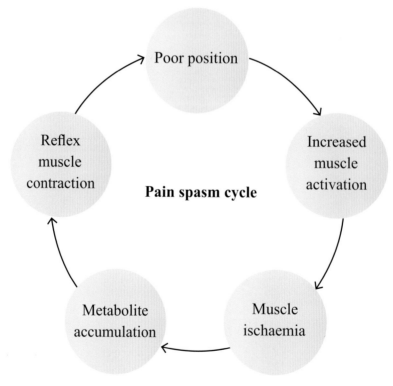

Figure 2.18: Pain spasm model.

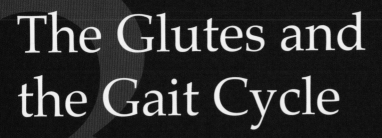

3

The Glutes and the Gait Cycle

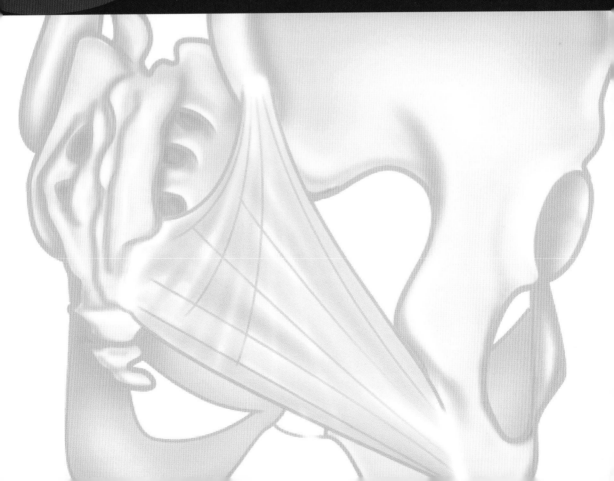

We take walking for granted—it is something that we just do without understanding what exactly is going on—until we suffer pain somewhere in our body, and then the simple action of walking becomes very painful. What I would like to do in this chapter is to discuss in detail what exactly happens when we walk (you might want to go through the movements yourself as they are described).

Gait Cycle

Definition: A *gait cycle* is a sequence of events in walking or running, beginning when one foot contacts the ground and ending when the same foot contacts the ground again.

The gait cycle is divided into two main phases: the *stance* phase and the *swing* phase. Each cycle begins at initial contact (also known as *heel-strike*) of the leading leg with a stance phase, proceeds through a swing phase, and ends with the next contact of the ground with that same leg. The stance phase is subdivided into *heel-strike*, *mid-stance*, and *propulsion* phases.

Human gait is a very complicated, coordinated series of movements. Another way of thinking about the gait cycle is that the stance phase is the weight-bearing component of each gait cycle. It is initiated by heel-strike and ends with toe-off from the same foot. The swing phase is initiated with toe-off and ends with heel-strike. It has been estimated that the stance phase accounts for approximately 60% of a single gait cycle, and the swing phase for approximately 40%.

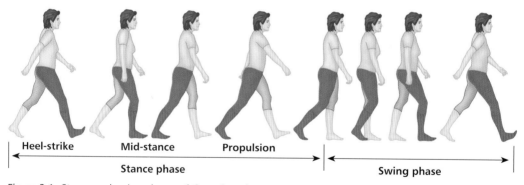

| Heel-strike | Mid-stance | Propulsion | | Swing phase |

Figure 3.1: Stance and swing phases of the gait cycle.

Heel-Strike

If you think about the position of your body just before you contact the ground with your right leg during the contact phase of the stance phase, the right hip is in a position of flexion, the knee is extended, the ankle is dorsiflexed, and the foot is in a position of supination. The tibialis anterior muscle, with the help of the tibialis posterior, works to maintain the ankle/foot in the position of dorsiflexion and inversion (inversion is part of the motion referred to as supination).

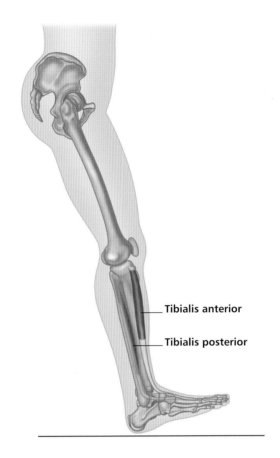

Tibialis anterior

Tibialis posterior

Figure 3.2: The position of the leg just before heel-strike.

In normal gait the foot strikes the ground at the beginning of the heel-strike in a supinated position of approximately 2 degrees. A normal foot will then move through 5–6 degrees of pronation at the subtalar joint (STJ) to a position of approximately 3–4 degrees of pronation, as this will allow the foot to function as a "mobile adaptor."

A Myofascial Link

As a result of the foot being dorsiflexed and supinated, the tibialis anterior (which is the main muscle responsible for this anatomical position and has an insertion on the medial cuneiform and 1st metatarsal) is now part of a link system that we will call a *myofascial sling*. This sling, starting from the initial origin of the tibialis anterior, continues as the insertion of the peroneus longus (onto the 1st metatarsal and medial cuneiform, as in the case of the tibialis anterior) to its muscular origin on the lateral side and head of the fibula. This bony landmark is also where the biceps femoris muscle inserts. The sling now continues as the biceps femoris muscle toward its origin on the ischial tuberosity, where the muscle attaches to the tuberosity via the sacrotuberous ligament; often the biceps femoris directly attaches to this ligament rather than to the ischial tuberosity, and some authors have mentioned that potentially 30% of the biceps femoris attaches directly to the inferior lateral angle (ILA) of the sacrum. The sling then carries on as the sacrotuberous ligament, which attaches to the inferior aspect of the sacrum at the ILA and fascially connects to the contralateral multifidi and to the erector spinae that continue to the base of the occipital bone. This myofascial sling is known as the *posterior longitudinal sling (PLS)*.

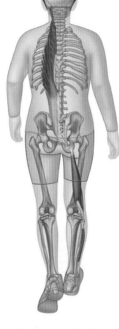

Figure 3.3: A person walking, with the posterior longitudinal muscles highlighted.

So even before you contact the ground, the posterior longitudinal sling is being fascially tensioned; the increased tension is focused on the sacrotuberous ligament via the attachment of the biceps femoris. This connection will assist the force closure mechanism process of the SIJ; in simple terms, this creates a stable pelvis for the initiation of the weight-bearing gait cycle. You may also notice that the right ilium (see figure 3.4) undergoes posterior rotation during the swing phase and this will assist the closure of the SIJ because of the increased tension of the sacrotuberous ligament.

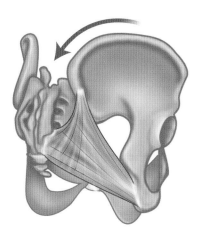

Figure 3.4: Right ilium in posterior rotation—sacrotuberous ligament tensioned.

You might want to stand and slowly go through the following movements so that you can get a sense of what happens with your body in normal walking. As explained above, just before the heel-strike phase your hip will be flexed, your knee extended, and your ankle dorsiflexed with the foot supinated. The tibialis anterior and tibialis posterior maintain this position of the ankle and foot, and as you contact the ground, these two muscles are responsible for controlling the rate of pronation through the STJ by contracting eccentrically.

As your right leg moves from heel-strike to toe-off, your body weight begins to move over your right leg, causing your pelvis to shift laterally to the right. As the movement continues toward toe-off, your right pelvic innominate bone begins to rotate anteriorly while your left innominate bone begins to rotate posteriorly.

As you continue with the gait cycle, you now enter the mid-stance phase of gait and this is where the hamstrings should reduce their tension by the natural anterior rotation of the pelvis and the slackening of the sacrotuberous ligament. This is the point during the mid-stance phase where the Gmax should take the role of extension.

Phasic contraction of the Gmax occurs in the mid-stance phase: the Gmax simultaneously contracts with the contralateral latissimus dorsi—it is this muscle that will extend the arm through what is known as *counterrotation*, to assist in propulsion. The thoracolumbar fascia, which is a sheet of connective tissue, is located between the Gmax and the contralateral latissimus dorsi, and this fascial structure is forced to increase its tension because of the contractions of the Gmax and latissimus dorsi. This increased tension will assist in stabilizing the SIJ of the stance leg through force closure.

If you look at figure 3.5 overleaf, you can see that just before heel-strike, the Gmax will reach maximum stretch as the latissimus dorsi is being stretched by the forward swing of the opposite arm. Heel-strike signifies a transition to the propulsive phase of gait, at which time the Gmax contraction is superimposed on that of the hamstrings.

Activation of the Gmax occurs in conjunction with contraction of the contralateral latissimus dorsi, which is now extending the arm in unison with the propelling leg. The synergistic contraction of the Gmax and latissimus dorsi creates tension in the thoracolumbar fascia, which will be released in a surge of energy that will assist the muscles of locomotion, reducing the overall energy expenditure of the gait cycle. Janda (1992, 1996) mentions that poor Gmax strength and activation is postulated to decrease the efficiency of gait.

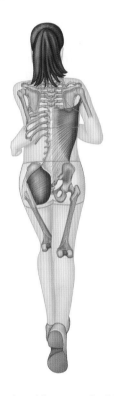

Figure 3.5: A person running, with the posterior oblique muscles highlighted.

As we progress from the mid-stance phase to heel-lift and propulsion, the foot begins to re-supinate and passes through a neutral position when the propulsive phase begins; the foot continues in supination through toe-off. As a result of the foot supinating during the mid-stance propulsive period, the foot is converted from a "mobile adaptor" (which is what it is during the contact period) to a "rigid lever" as the mid-tarsal joint locks into a supinated position. With the foot functioning as a rigid lever (as a result of the locked mid-tarsal joint) during the time immediately preceding toe-off, the weight of the body is propelled more efficiently.

Pelvis Motion

Next we will take a look at the pelvis and how it functions during the mid-stance phase. As the right innominate bone starts to rotate anteriorly from an initial posterior rotated position, the sacrum will be forced to move into what is called a *right torsion on the right oblique axis (R on R)*. In other words, the sacrum rotates to the right, and side bends to the left, because the left sacral base moves into an anterior nutation position (this is also known as *Type I spinal mechanics*, as the rotation and side-bending are coupled to opposite sides) as shown is figure 3.6a. Owing to the kinematics of the sacrum, the lumbar spine rotates left and side bends to the right as shown is figure 3.6b, the thoracic spine rotates right and side bends to the left, and the cervical spine rotates right and side bends to the right. The cervical spine coupling is opposite to that of the other vertebrae since its spinal mechanics are Type II (Type II means that rotation and side-bending are coupled to the same side). As the left leg moves from weight bearing to toe-off, the left innominate, the sacrum, and the lumbar and thoracic vertebrae undergo torsion, rotation, and side-bending in a similar manner to that described above, but with movements in the opposite directions.

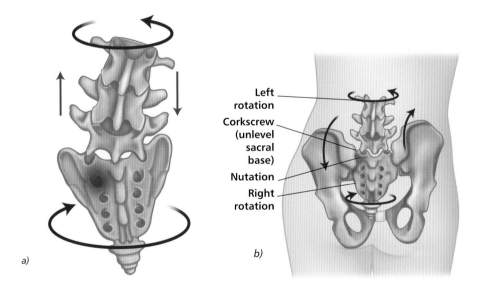

Left rotation

Corkscrew (unlevel sacral base)

Nutation

Right rotation

a)

b)

Figure 3.6: Sacral rotation and lumbar counterrotation.

The anterior oblique also works in conjunction with the stance leg adductors, ipsilateral internal oblique, and contralateral external oblique muscles, as shown in figure 3.7. These integrated muscle contractions help stabilize the body on top of the stance leg and assist in rotating the pelvis forward for optimum propulsion in preparation for the ensuing heel-strike.

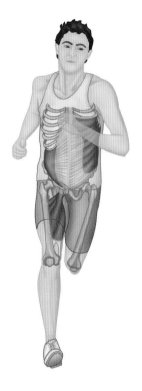

Figure 3.7: A person running, with anterior sling muscles highlighted.

The swing phase of gait utilizes the lateral system, as we have entered the single-leg stance position. This sling connects the gluteus medius (Gmed) and gluteus minimus (Gmin) of the stance leg, and the ipsilateral adductors, with the contralateral quadratus lumborum (QL). Contraction of the left Gmed and adductors stabilizes the pelvis, and activation of the contralateral QL will assist in elevation of the pelvis; this will allow enough lift of the pelvis to permit the leg to go through the swing phase of gait. The lateral sling plays a critical role, as it assists in stabilizing the spine and hip joints in the frontal plane and is a necessary contributor to the overall stability of the pelvis and trunk.

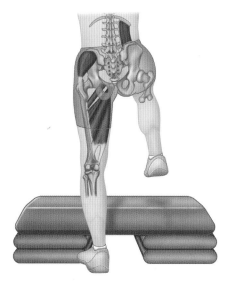

Figure 3.8: A step-up indicates an example of the swing phase of gait, with lateral sling muscles highlighted.

Maitland (2001) mentions that proper body movement while walking is influenced by the ability of the sacrum to cope with left torsion on the left oblique axis (L on L) and right torsion on the right oblique axis (R on R). Since most walking is accomplished with your vertebral column relatively upright and vertical, for the purpose of this discussion we will assume that your spine and sacrum are in neutral while you walk.

The way our axial skeletal system alternately undulates in side-bending and rotation as we walk is very interesting and extremely important to our overall well-being. It is a movement that is reminiscent of the undulating action of a snake as it slithers through the grass. The big difference between a snake and a human, of course, is that our snakelike spine has ended up being given two legs on which to walk.

4
Leg Length Discrepancy and Over-Pronation —the Effect on the Glutes

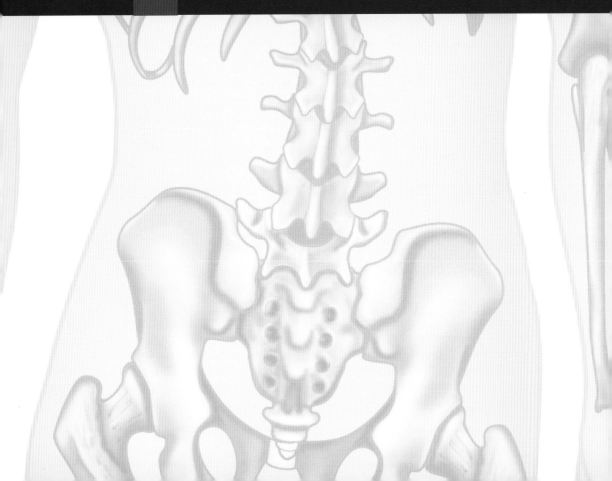

The majority of patients visiting my clinic present with pain somewhere in their bodies. Part of my initial assessment is to have the patient stand with their back to me; with them in this position, I place both my hands on top of their iliac crest to see if there is any pelvic obliquity, in other words a low or a high side, as shown in figure 4.1. Very often I do find that there is a discrepancy in the level of the height of the iliac crest between the two sides, which could possibly indicate a leg length discrepancy (LLD), or, as it has been alternatively termed, a *short leg syndrome* or a *long leg syndrome*. LLD is possibly the most significant postural asymmetry that presents itself to the physical therapist. The existence of a considerable difference between the two sides can be very detrimental to how we function on a day-to-day basis as well as during the gait cycle: the discrepancy can significantly affect our overall posture.

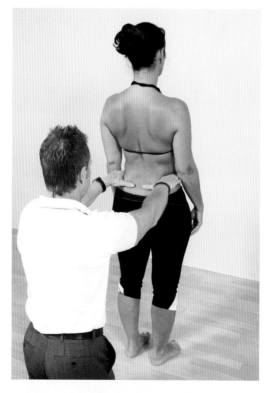

Figure 4.1: Measurement of leg length by palpation of the iliac crest.

Definition: *Leg length discrepancy (LLD)* is a condition where one leg is shorter than the other.

One has to decide if there is an "actual" (or "true") leg length discrepancy or an "apparent" leg length discrepancy, as LLD has been implicated in all sorts of deficiency related our gait and running mechanics. LLD has also been linked to postural dysfunctions, as well as to increased incidence of scoliosis, lower back and sacroiliac pain, and osteoarthritis (OA) of the hip and knee. Even stress fractures of the hip, spine, and lower extremity have been related to changes in leg length.

The *actual* (true) leg length measurement is the length that is typically determined by the use of a tape measure from a point on the pelvis—the anterior superior iliac spine (ASIS)—to the medial malleolus, as shown in figure 4.2; the ASIS is normally used as the landmark, since it is impossible to palpate the femur below the iliac crest. Before taking this measurement, it is beneficial to measure the distance from the ASIS on the left and right sides to the umbilicus, as shown in figure 4.3, to ascertain if any pelvic rotation is present. If a difference in the two measurements is found, the pelvic rotations need to be corrected before a reassessment is done.

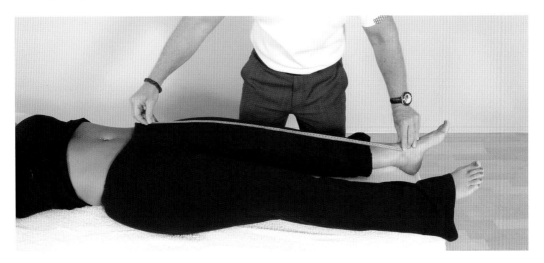

Figure 4.2: True leg length measurement, taken from the ASIS to the medial malleolus.

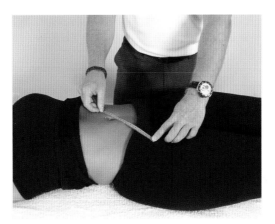

Figure 4.3: Measurement taken from the ASIS to the umbilicus.

If the measurements taken from the ASIS to the medial malleolus on both sides are the same, it can then be assumed that the length of each limb is equal; on the other hand, if the measurements differ, one can assume that an actual leg length discrepancy is present.

The *apparent* leg length measurement is taken from the umbilicus to the medial malleolus, as shown in figure 4.4. If the measurements taken on both sides are different, one can assume that a dysfunction exists somewhere which will require further investigation.

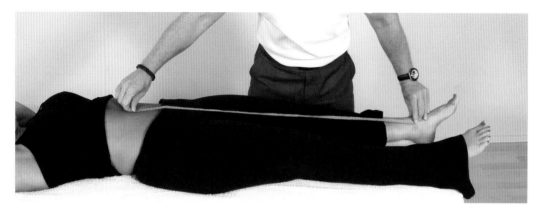

Figure 4.4: Apparent leg length measurement, taken from the umbilicus to the medial malleolus.

Types of LLD

LLD can be divided into three main groups:

1. **Structural:** This is an actual (or true) shortening of the skeletal system, typically caused by one of four things:
   - Congenital defect, e.g. congenital dysplasia of the hip joint
   - Surgery, e.g. total hip replacement (THR)
   - Trauma, e.g. fractured femur or tibia
   - Disease process, e.g. tumor, arthritis, or Perthes disease

   Fractured bones in children have been known to grow faster for many years after the healing process: this can naturally result in the limb becoming anatomically longer.

2. **Functional:** This can be a development from altered biomechanics of the lower body, such as ankle and foot over-pronation or supination, pelvic obliquity, muscle imbalances (as a result of, for instance, a weak Gmed or tight adductors), hip or knee joint dysfunction, and even poor inner core stabilization, to name a few.

3. **Idiopathic:** If there are obvious findings during the history taking and assessment process, the physical therapist may have an idea as to the cause of the patient's LLD. However, if the therapist cannot ascertain a reason for the change in the presenting leg length, the condition would be classified as *idiopathic*, which means that it arises independently, not as a result of some other condition.

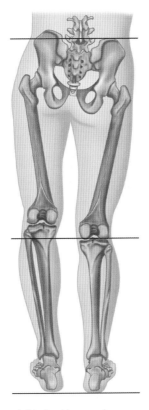

Figure 4.5: Left long leg syndrome versus right short leg syndrome.

Assessment

The therapist has to be very intuitive during the initial assessment. When the iliac crest is palpated on a patient in a standing position, the therapist needs to be aware of a "pelvic shift" as the patient stands. Let me give you an example: if the patient has a weak Gmed muscle on the left, the pelvis will appear to drop to the right and deviate or laterally shift to the left, which will cause the left iliac crest to appear elevated on that side (left), giving the appearance of a longer left leg.

When the patient presents to the clinic, we can assume that the pain has existed for a while, and so we can say that it is at the chronic stage. Because of the natural overcompensatory mechanisms that occur through chronicity, the postural muscles are probably held in a shortened and subsequently tight position; one muscle in particular that has a tendency to shorten is the QL. A problem can arise when the patient lies on their back (supine position) so that you can observe the positions of the left and right medial malleoli when looking for any leg length discrepancy. You may now notice that the left medial malleolus is nearer to the patient's head than the one on the right, giving the appearance of a short left leg as a result of a tight left QL. When the patient was standing, however, you may have convinced yourself that the patient's left leg looked longer!

This might initially seem confusing, but just think about it for a moment. Could it not simply mean that when the patient adopts a standing position the Gmed on the left side is weak, causing the pelvis to shift to the side of weakness? Conversely, is it not possible that when the patient is in a supine position, the left QL is held in a shortened position, which is responsible for hitching up the pelvis, having the effect of pulling the leg closer to the head and thus making the leg appear shorter?

When you are standing, the *weak* muscles show themselves; when you are lying, the *short* muscles show themselves.

Foot and Ankle Position

One of the most neglected aspects of the body when patients present to the clinic is the position of the lower limb. Osteopaths, chiropractors, and physical therapists see lots of patients who initially present with lower back and sacroiliac pain. These specialist therapists naturally spend a lot of time observing and assessing the pelvis and lumbar spine to ascertain which tissue is giving the person the pain. This presenting pain may, however, just be a symptom, and the cause of the pain could be somewhere else, away from the actual site of the pain.

The only person interested in the pain is your patient; you the therapist should try to find the cause of the pain and not treat where it simply hurts.

It is very important that when assessing your patients you observe the position of the lower limb and in particular the foot and ankle complex, as a faulty foot and ankle structure can profoundly affect leg length and the natural position of the pelvis. The most common asymmetrical foot position that patients present with has to be what is commonly called an *over-pronated foot*, as shown in figure 4.6. It has been widely thought that when we actually present with a true leg length discrepancy, the body will try to compensate for the longer leg through lowering the medial arch of the foot by pronating at the STJ. The action of pronation is called *tri-planar motion* and consists of three movements: dorsiflexion of the ankle, eversion, and abduction of the foot complex. The position of this increased pronation is basically the body's natural compensatory mechanism to try to "shorten" the leg because it is anatomically longer.

The plantar surface of our feet has thousands of sensory receptors that are responsible for the position of the foot; the smallest shift in weight will be enough to signal the brain to induce a compensatory reaction. On the contralateral side (shorter leg), the compensatory mechanism will cause the medial arch to adopt a supinated position (tri-planar motion of plantar flexion, inversion, and adduction). The compensatory mechanism changes the position of the arch in an attempt to lengthen the apparent shorter leg. When physical therapists assess their patients they will need to check for this compensatory pattern, because, if left unchecked, excessive foot pronation caused by an anatomically longer leg (subsequent supination of the contralateral foot as compensation) will in turn cause an internal rotation of the lower extremity and contralateral external rotation. This will then have the effect of altering the whole kinetic chain from the foot all the way up to the occiput.

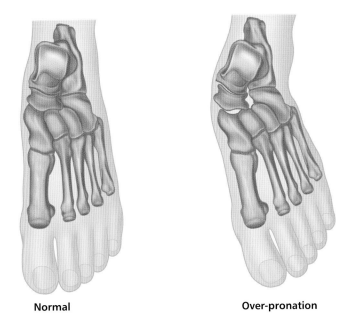

Normal   **Over-pronation**

Figure 4.6: Over-pronation syndrome.

True LLD and the Relationship to the Pelvis

Let's continue with a "thought process" just for a moment. Now consider that your patient has a longer leg on the left side, which you have ascertained because of the higher position of the iliac crest and the possible compensatory pronation of the STJ on the same side. Before I continue with the discussion, just have a think to yourself about what position the innominate bone might be in if the left leg, say, is anatomically longer.

The innominate rotation will naturally be coupled with a leg length discrepancy as a result of the compensatory mechanisms: if you look at figure 4.7 overleaf, you will see that the femoral head on the long-leg side forces the innominate into a superior and posteriorly rotated position. Conversely, the innominate on the low femoral head side drops down and anteriorly rotates, as shown in figure 4.8 overleaf. What we have now, therefore, is the left innominate being forced into a posterior rotation and the right innominate into an anterior rotation. Think about what lies between the two innominates—yes, the sacrum bone. As a result of the compensatory rotation of both of the innominate bones in opposite directions to each other, a motion of the sacrum occurs, known in osteopathic terms as a *left-on-left (L-on-L) sacral torsion* (figure 4.9 overleaf). An L-on-L sacral torsion means that the sacrum has rotated to the left on the left oblique axis and has side bent to the right, as it is ruled by Type I spinal mechanics (rotation and side-bending are coupled to opposite sides, as established by Fryette (1918) and the law of spinal mechanics). This complexity which has been described of the innominate rotations that are coupled with a sacral torsion is usually depicted as a *pelvic torsion*, or even a *pelvic obliquity*, and will require a good understanding before a treatment plan is introduced.

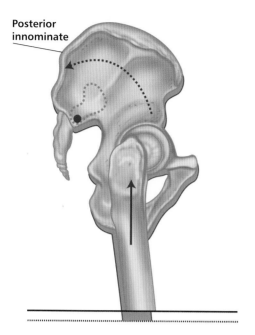

Posterior innominate

Figure 4.7: Long leg innominate compensation.

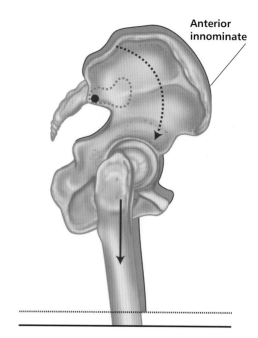

Anterior innominate

Figure 4.8: Short leg innominate compensation.

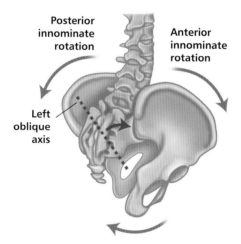

Posterior innominate rotation

Anterior innominate rotation

Left oblique axis

Figure 4.9: L-on-L sacral torsion.

True LLD and the Relationship between the Trunk and the Head

You will notice in figure 4.10 that on the left side there is a lower shoulder position on the high innominate side: this is a common finding in the case of a compensatory functional scoliosis. Some authors, however, have considered this to occur as a result of a "handedness pattern": for example, if you are left handed, the left shoulder might appear to be lower, and if you are right handed, the right shoulder might appear to be lower.

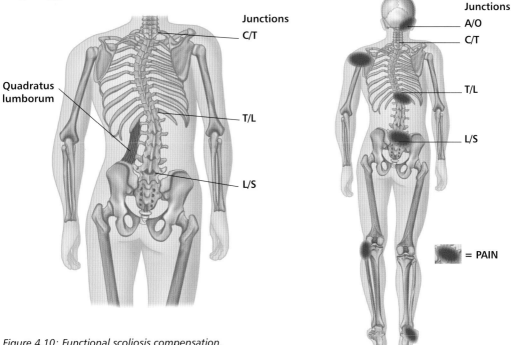

Figure 4.10: Functional scoliosis compensation.

What else do you observe in figure 4.10? If you look at what is happening to the left quadratus lumborum, you would assume that this muscle is being held in a shortened position because of the higher left innominate. This assumption is correct, as you can also see that the lumbar spine is side bending toward the longer left leg and rotating toward the shorter right leg.

As a result of the ascending functional scoliosis, the right shoulder is higher. You might also notice a short "C" curve in the cervical spine; this will probably cause the scalenes, SCM, upper trapezius, and possibly the levator scapulae muscles on the right side to adopt a shortened and subsequently tight position. This typical adaptation of muscular imbalance will help maintain an erect head position with the eyes level. The body will always want to be level no matter what and will do almost anything to accomplish this, including enduring pain to maintain equilibrium. Common painful conditions that patients might present with are headaches, active trigger points, tinnitus, temporomandibular joint (TMJ) dysfunction, and even eye and facial pain.

LLD and the Gait Cycle

As we walk, if our gait cycle pattern has been altered because of an actual or an apparent LLD, the shorter leg will feel like it is stepping down, and the long leg will compensate by a sort of "vaulting" motion. It is almost like stepping into a small pothole with every step you take; imagine repeating this at least ten to fifteen thousand times a day—it will easily cause potential pain patterns of dysfunction! Common compensations are sometimes seen when patients are asked to walk: on the short-leg side, the patient might have a tendency to walk on their toes, and on the long-leg side, the patient may have a tendency to flex their knee, but this will depend on the discrepancy.

For the body to be an effective locomotor during the gait cycle, a well-aligned and symmetrical body is essential. When the positions of the innominate bones of the pelvis are altered by actual or apparent leg length discrepancies, it is easy to see how patients can present with pain, not only at the sacroiliac joint and lumbar spine but also everywhere else in their body that is going through a compensation pattern.

I mentioned earlier that there could be a weakness of the Gmed on one side of the body, and a shortness issue with the tensor fasciae latae (TFL) and iliotibial band (ITB) on the other side. If there is weakness of the Gmed, the patient can have either a *Trendelenburg* pattern of gait or a *compensatory Trendelenburg* pattern of gait (this is explained in more detail in chapter 6). Whichever way you look at this, the patient is going to have an antalgic type of gait, which simply means that they will walk with some form of limp; this compensation can only cause one thing over time and that will simply be pain.

Summary of Compensations to the Iliopsoas

- The iliopsoas muscle is generally tight on the side of the short leg. Note that a left iliopsoas muscle spasm will cause a pelvic side shift to the right, mimicking a short left leg.
- The innominate bone may compensate by rotating anteriorly on the side of the short leg, functionally lengthening that leg, while the innominate on the long side may do the opposite.
- Unilateral spasm of the iliopsoas creates lumbar concavity on the opposite side and sets up a positive side shift on the side opposite to the spasm. It is important that the physical therapist always assess for and treat iliopsoas spasm in the case of a suspected short leg or a positive pelvic lateral side shift.
- Iliopsoas spasm pain is worse on standing from a seated position, and less pain is perceived as the iliopsoas stretches out.

Summary of Compensations to the Sacrum and Lumbar Spine

- Sacrum typically rotates toward the long leg and side bends toward the short leg.
- Posterior sacrum might be associated with same-side piriformis spasm.
- Anterior sacrum might be associated with same-side Gmed spasm.
- Lumbar spine typically side bends to the long-leg side and rotates toward the side of the low sacral base/short leg.
- Facet pain due to compression is common on the concavity side of the lumbar spine.
- Iliolumbar ligament can cause pain as it is stretched on the convex side of the lumbar spine and has been argued to refer pain to the groin, testicle, and medial thigh on the same side as the stretched ligament.

In summary, when looking at the level of the iliac crest, one has to determine if there is a leg length discrepancy. If there is, one then has to ascertain if the dysfunction is a true discrepancy or a functional discrepancy, as the compensation pattern can change depending on the diagnosis. For example, if you find a true anatomical leg length discrepancy, the innominate bone on the longer leg will try to compensate by rotating posteriorly, as seen in figure 4.7 and explained earlier. Moreover, the femur and lower limb on the anatomically longer leg will follow the compensatory model by rotating medially, as seen in figure 4.5, and the foot will try to pronate at the STJ, since the longer leg will attempt to *shorten* itself. At the same time, the actual shorter leg will compensate by supinating at the ankle mortise; this in effect can cause the tibia and femur to rotate externally and the innominate bone to rotate anteriorly as the leg tries to make itself appear *longer.*

Over-Pronation Syndrome

Let's look at another compensation model for a patient who appears to have a leg length discrepancy. In this case it is a functional LLD, and the apparent shorter leg of the patient exhibits an over-pronation of the STJ, rather than the longer leg compensating by pronating to shorten itself. As a result, the body will try to compensate by causing an internal rotation of the tibia and femur (figure 4.11); this will have the effect of the innominate bone rotating anteriorly, which in turn can cause an increased lumbar lordosis with subsequent lower back pain.

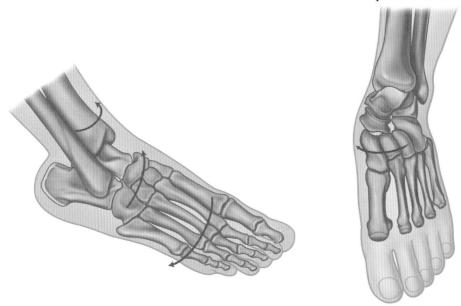

Figure 4.11: A foot in over-pronation with internal tibial rotation.

Over-pronation is a common pattern found in the majority of people to some extent or another. It is best identified with the patient standing barefoot. The big clue is that one arch is lower or flatter than the other: the lower arch side is over-pronating. Sometimes, both sides may be over-pronating, but one side is generally over-pronating more than the other, or one side might be normal and the other side lower. It is easy to confirm the condition by simply placing one finger under the patient's arch, noting how much of your finger goes underneath, and comparing the result with the other side. Are they the same or different? If one side is noticeably lower than the other, you have found a patient with an over-pronation syndrome. Another test to confirm over-pronation is to observe the Achilles tendon from the posterior aspect: you will typically notice a bowing on the side with the lower arch.

It should be noted that over-pronation syndrome can originate not only from the foot and ankle but also from the innominate of that side. When the foot and ankle complex over-pronates, the innominate bone will normally rotate anteriorly. However, if we look at it from the other way around, an anterior rotation of the innominate can force the medial arch of the foot into an over-pronated position. This becomes a chicken and the egg situation, but that is irrelevant, as the only consideration is whatever presents itself now. In my experience, you might need to correct the innominate's rotation and the over-pronation to help reduce the patient's presenting symptoms.

You can see already that both compensatory mechanisms have a pronation issue at the STJ; however, the true leg length compensation of the longer leg forced the innominate bone to rotate *posteriorly*, whereas the functional leg length discrepancy of the over-pronation syndrome caused the innominate bone to rotate *anteriorly*.

You can probably gather from all the information above that there can be so much going on at the same time throughout the kinetic chain; everything that has been mentioned can affect the *length* of the leg. It is correct to assume that this area of discussion is somewhat complex, and it might be difficult to know where to start in the assessment or even in the treatment program.

In all that has been discussed above, there lies a potential solution to the jigsaw puzzle of patients' symptoms and dysfunctions. There exists what I call a *key* to unlocking the problem; the difficulty in physical therapy, however, is finding where to start and "insert the key" (excuse the expression). I can guarantee that, over the years, inexperienced therapists will have time and time again inserted the key into the wrong place, i.e. where the patient feels the pain and not where the problem lies. Recall the wise words of Dr. Ida Rolf!

When I teach physical therapists today, sometimes during the practical sessions I say "Treat what you find"; the body will hopefully guide them onto the correct pathway. If, after three or even four physical therapy sessions, a patient's symptoms are not reducing, then you the therapist will need to change your thought process and treat other areas that you initially felt might not be related to the cause of the patient's presenting pain patterns.

LLD and the Glutes

So how does all this affect the glutes? When you have a compensation pattern, the femur not only rotates to compensate in the transverse plane, but also experiences a compensatory mechanism of adduction and abduction in the frontal plane. Thus, in simple terms, if you have a lower limb that is held in an adducted position then the abductor muscle group can be forced into a lengthened and subsequently weakened position, while the adductors will be held in a shortened and subsequently tight position. For a leg that is held in abduction, the situation is reversed.

If you look back at figure 4.5 you will see that the left leg appears longer because of the higher left iliac crest, the innominate has rotated posteriorly, the femur has internally rotated, and the foot has pronated. In this compensation the left leg will be in a position of adduction (figure 4.12), and consequently the right leg will be held in a position of abduction (figure 4.13). This will have an effect on the musculature of the associated areas: some of these muscles will be held in a shortened position and some in a lengthened position.

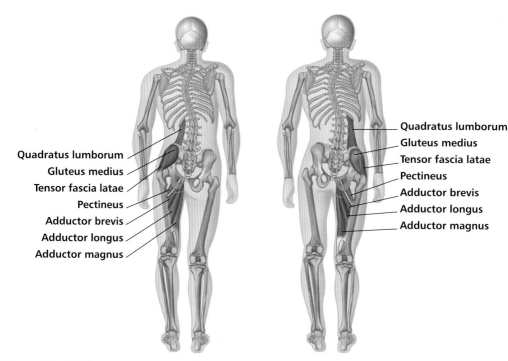

Figure 4.12: Left leg compensations—adductors and QL short and tight, with Gmed and TFL long and weak.

Figure 4.13: Right leg compensations—adductors and QL long and weak, with Gmed and TFL short and tight.

Standing Balance Test

When a patient is asked to stand on one leg and lift the opposite knee toward their waist, the physical therapist needs to observe the level of the PSIS as the patient transfers their weight to one leg. The patient should be able to shift their weight onto the stance leg (the right leg in figure 4.14), with good muscular control of the Gmed of that leg. If the PSIS dips down on the leg that is being lifted (the left leg in figure 4.14) rather than remaining level, it might be assumed that the Gmed on the other side is unable to control the movement; the patient might then have an altered pattern of gait when they go through the gait cycle, as shown in figure 4.15. This altered gait pattern is called a *Trendelenburg gait* and is illustrated for a weak left Gmed in figure 4.16. If this dysfunctional gait is present over a prolonged period, a compensatory Trendelenburg might develop, as shown in figure 4.17. The reasons for this altered gait can be numerous to say the least, but one cause could be that one of the legs is held in an adducted position because of the shortening of the adductors (as mentioned above). This altered pattern will in turn result in a reciprocal inhibition: the abductors—in particular the Gmed—will now be held in a lengthened position that can then predispose the Gmed to becoming weak.

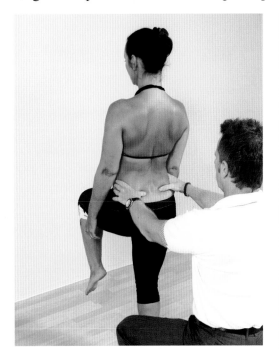

Figure 4.14: Standing balance test—normal.

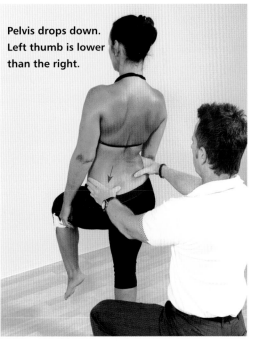

Pelvis drops down. Left thumb is lower than the right.

Figure 4.15: Positive test for weakness of the right Gmed—the PSIS dips down on the left.

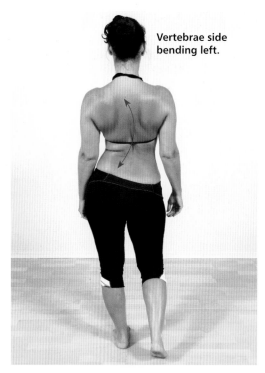
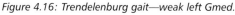
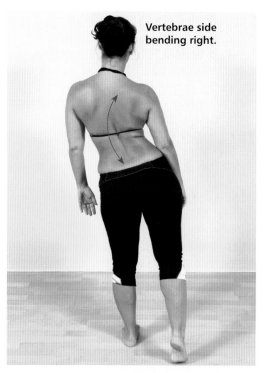

Vertebrae side bending left.

Vertebrae side bending right.

Figure 4.16: Trendelenburg gait—weak left Gmed.

Figure 4.17: Compensatory Trendelenburg gait— weak left Gmed.

When I teach the standing balance test (figure 4.14), I say to my students that you need to look out for three things. The first, as I mentioned above, is the position of the PSIS as the patient transfers their weight from one leg to the other. The second is how much movement occurs as the patient shifts onto the weight-bearing leg; you may notice one side shifting more than the other, indicating a possible Gmed weakness. Finally, the third is how stable the patient is when they stand on one leg compared with the other. You will be amazed how many very fit athletes struggle to stand on one leg unaided and maintain good control.

Hopefully, after reading this chapter, you will have some understanding of what is happening when a patient presents with musculoskeletal dysfunctions, such as leg length discrepancy, over-pronation syndrome, and muscle imbalances. In the next chapter I will continue with the journey on this theme by looking at the functional anatomy of the Gmax. Then, in chapter 6, we will look more closely at the function of the Gmed and how it can alter our gait patterns.

Functional Anatomy of the Gluteus Maximus

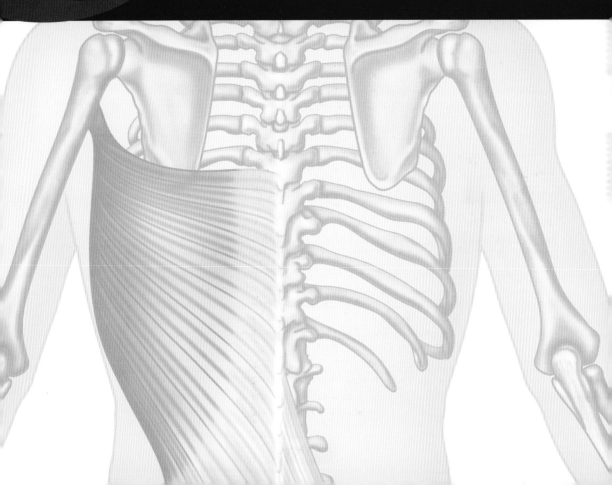

This chapter will focus on the gluteus maximus (Gmax) and how this muscle could be responsible for many of the complaints that patients and athletes present with, especially painful symptoms in the area of the lower back. The Gmax, I feel, is relatively neglected by most physical therapists I come into contact with. Perhaps the reason for this neglect is that the Gmax does not normally itself present with pain, and hence this amazing and functional muscle is left on what I call the *neglect shelf*.

Gmax Anatomy

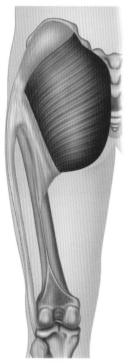

Origin
Outer surface of the ilium behind the posterior gluteal line and a portion of the bone superior and posterior to it. Adjacent posterior surface of the sacrum and coccyx. Sacrotuberous ligament. Aponeurosis of the erector spinae.

Insertion
Deep fibers of distal portion: Gluteal tuberosity of the femur.
Remaining fibers: Iliotibial tract of the fasciae latae.

Action
Assists in adduction of hip joint. Through its insertion into the iliotibial tract, helps to stabilize the knee in extension.
Upper fibers: Laterally rotate and may assist in abduction of hip joint.
Lower fibers: Extend and laterally rotate hip joint (forceful extension as in running or standing up from sitting). Extend trunk.

Nerve
Inferior gluteal nerve (L5, S1, S2).

Figure 5.1: Origin, insertion, action, and nerve innervation of the Gmax.

Function of the Gmax

From a functional perspective, the Gmax performs several key roles in controlling the relationship between the pelvis, trunk, and femur. This muscle is capable of abducting and laterally rotating the hip, which helps to control the alignment of the knee with the lower limb. For example, in stair climbing, the Gmax will laterally rotate and abduct the hip to keep the lower limb in optimal alignment, while at the same time the hip extends to carry the body upward onto the next step. When the Gmax is weak or misfiring, the knee can be seen to deviate medially and the pelvis can also be observed to tip laterally.

The Gmax also has a role in stabilizing the SIJs and has been described as one of the force closure muscles. Some of the Gmax fibers attach to the sacrotuberous ligament and the thoracolumbar fascia, which is a very strong, non-contractile connective tissue that is tensioned by the activation of muscles connecting to it. One of the connections to this fascia is the latissimus dorsi. The Gmax forms a partnership with the contralateral latissimus dorsi via the thoracolumbar fascia— this partnership connection is known as the *posterior oblique sling* (see figure 5.2). This sling increases the compression force to the SIJ during the weight-bearing single-leg stance in the gait cycle.

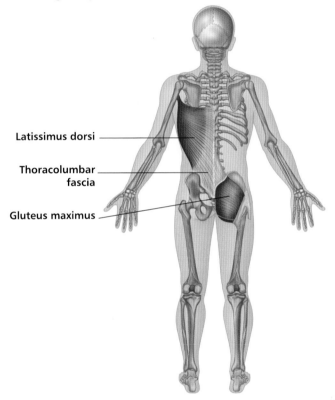

Latissimus dorsi

Thoracolumbar fascia

Gluteus maximus

Figure 5.2: Posterior oblique sling and the connection with the latissimus dorsi.

Misfiring or weakness in the Gmax reduces the effectiveness of the posterior oblique sling, which will predispose the SIJs to subsequent injury. The body will then try to compensate for this weakness by increasing tension via the thoracolumbar fascia by in turn increasing the activation of the contralateral latissimus dorsi. As with any compensatory mechanism, "structure affects function" and "function affects structure." This means that other areas of the body are affected: for example, the shoulder mechanics are altered since the latissimus dorsi has attachments on the humerus and scapula. If the latissimus dorsi is particularly active because of the compensation, this can be observed as one shoulder appearing lower than the other during a step-up or a lunge type of motion.

As explained in chapter 3, the Gmax plays a significant role in the gait cycle, working in conjunction with the hamstrings. Just before heel-strike, the hamstrings will activate, which will increase the tension to the SIJs via the attachment on the sacrotuberous ligament. This connection assists in the locking mechanism of the SIJs for the weight-bearing cycle. From heel-strike to mid-stance of the gait cycle, the Gmax increases its activation and the hamstrings decrease theirs. The Gmax significantly increases the stabilization of the SIJs during early and mid-stance phases through the attachments of the posterior oblique sling.

Weakness or misfiring in the Gmax will cause the hamstrings to remain active during the gait cycle in order to maintain stability of the SIJs and the position of the pelvis. The resultant overactivation of the hamstrings will subject them to continual and abnormal strain.

As I said earlier, the focus of this chapter is to look at what happens when the Gmax is involved. Generally the Gmax follows a trait of becoming weakened if the antagonistic muscles have become short and tight. However, the Gmax can also test weak if there is a neurological disorder affecting the L5 and S1 nerve root (which innervates the Gmax muscle), in turn having an impact on muscle contraction. This aspect will be discussed in greater detail in chapter 11.

The main muscles that can cause a neurological inhibition to the Gmax are the iliopsoas, rectus femoris, and adductors, as they all are classified as *hip flexors*, which are the antagonistic muscles to the hip extension action of the Gmax.

The assessment of the iliopsoas and other associated shortened antagonistic muscles will be discussed in chapter 8. Once that assessment has been fully understood, I will then teach you how to normalize the tight and shortened antagonistic muscles by the use of myofascial and muscle energy techniques. After mastering these advanced techniques, the physical therapist will be able to incorporate them into their own treatment modality with the aim of encouraging the lengthening of the tight tissues. This will then promote a normal neutral position of the pelvis and lumbar spine, and in turn hopefully have the effect of "switching" the weakened Gmax back on.

Assessment of the Gmax

In this section I will discuss the hip extension firing pattern test, which is used for determining the correct firing order of the hip extensors (including the Gmax muscle). The aim of the test is to ascertain the actual firing sequence of a group of muscles to ensure that all are firing correctly, just like the cylinders of an engine. A misfiring pattern will commonly be found in athletes and patients.

Hip Extension Firing Pattern Test

Figure 5.3 shows the correct firing pattern of hip joint extension. The normal muscle activation sequence is:

1. Gluteus maximus
2. Hamstrings
3. Contralateral lumbar extensors
4. Ipsilateral lumbar extensors
5. Contralateral thoracolumbar extensors
6. Ipsilateral thoracolumbar extensors

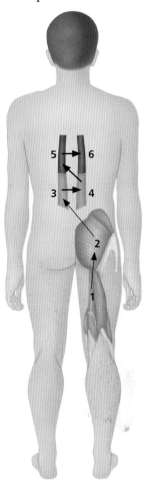

Muscle activation sequence

1. Hamstrings
2. Gluteus maximus

Either group may normally activate first

3. Contralateral lumbar extensors
4. Ipsilateral lumbar extensors
5. Contralateral thoracolumbar extensors
6. Ipsilateral thoracolumbar extensors

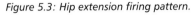

Figure 5.3: Hip extension firing pattern.

The hip extension firing pattern test is unique in its application. Think of yourself as a car with six cylinders in your engine: basically that is what your body is—an engine. The engine has a certain way of firing and so does your body. For example, the engine in a car will not fire its individual cylinders in the numerical order 1–2–3–4–5–6; it will fire in a pre-defined optimum sequence, say 1–3–5–6–4–2. If we have our car serviced and the mechanic mistakes two of the leads and puts them back incorrectly, the engine will still work but not very efficiently; moreover, it will eventually break down. Our bodies are no different: in our case, if we are particularly active but have a misfiring dysfunction, our bodies will also break down, ultimately causing us pain.

Sequence 1

The therapist places their fingertips lightly on the patient's left hamstrings and left Gmax (figures 5.4(a) and (b)), and the patient is asked to lift their left leg 2" (5 cm) off the couch (figure 5.4(c)). The therapist tries to identify which muscle fires first and notes the result of this first sequence in table 5.1.

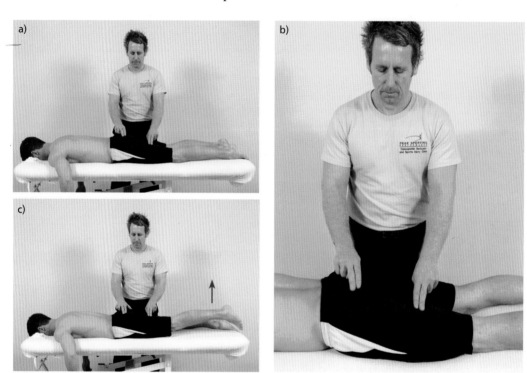

Figure 5.4: Hip extension firing pattern—sequence 1: (a) The therapist lightly palpates the patient's left hamstrings and Gmax; (b) Close-up view of the therapist's hand position; (c) The patient lifts their left leg off the couch.

Sequence 2

The therapist places their thumbs lightly on the patient's erector spinae, and the patient is asked to lift their left leg 2" off the couch (figure 5.5(a) and (b)). The therapist identifies and notes in table 5.1 which erector muscle fires first.

a)
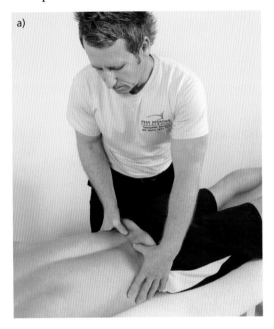

b)
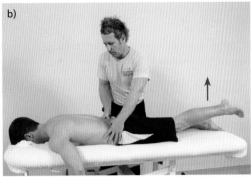

Figure 5.5: Hip extension firing pattern—sequence 2: (a) The therapist lightly palpates the patient's erector spinae; (b) The patient lifts their left leg off the couch.

	1st	**2nd**	**3rd**	**4th**
Gluteus maximus	○	○	○	○
Hamstrings	○	○	○	○
Contralateral erector spinae	○	○	○	○
Ipsilateral erector spinae	○	○	○	○

Table 5.1: Hip extension firing pattern—left side.

	1st	**2nd**	**3rd**	**4th**
Gluteus maximus	○	○	○	○
Hamstrings	○	○	○	○
Contralateral erector spinae	○	○	○	○
Ipsilateral erector spinae	○	○	○	○

Table 5.2: Hip extension firing pattern—right side.

Sequences 1 and 2 are then repeated with the right leg and the results recorded in table 5.2. Having done this, the therapist can determine whether or not the muscles are firing correctly. The firing pattern should be: (1) gluteus maximus; (2) hamstrings; (3) contralateral erector spinae; and, lastly, (4) ipsilateral erector spinae.

If, when palpating in sequence 1, the gluteus maximus is found to fire first, you can safely say that this is correct. The same applies in sequence 2: if the contralateral erector spinae contracts first, this is also the correct sequence.

However, if you feel that the hamstrings are number 1 in the sequence, or that the ipsilateral erector spinae is number 1 and the gluteus maximus is not felt to contract, you can deduce that this is a misfiring pattern. If the misfiring dysfunction is not corrected, our body (the engine) will start to break down and a compensatory pattern of dysfunction will be created.

In my experience I have found that in a lot of patients, the hamstrings and the ipsilateral erector spinae are typically first to contract and the Gmax is number four in the sequence. In these cases the erector spinae and the hamstrings will become the dominant muscles in assisting the hip in an extension movement. This can cause excessive anterior tilting of the pelvis with a resultant hyperlordosis, which can lead to inflammation of the lower lumbar facet joints. To correct the misfiring sequence, we need to look at chapter 8 on muscle length testing and the use of METs and myofascial techniques to treat and normalize shortened and tight tissues.

Note that the firing patterns of muscles 5 and 6 have not been discussed in this chapter, because we need to make sure that the correct firing order of muscles 1–4 is established. I also find that when the muscle 1–4 firing sequence has been corrected, the firing pattern of muscles 5 and 6 is generally self-correcting and tends to follow the normal firing pattern sequence.

Case Study

I have had the good fortune to be the sports osteopath looking after the Oxford University Boat Club for several years, particularly in preparation for the annual boat race against Cambridge University. During those years you can imagine how many of the rowers I have assessed and treated. One of the most common complaints that a rower presents to me at my sports injury clinic is lower back pain. This type of pain can include a multitude of pathologies that include facet joint syndrome, lower lumbar disc bulge, iliolumbar ligament sprain, multifidi strain—the list goes on and on.

Before rushing in to treat the area of pain, the physical therapist should ask themselves the following question: Is the patient's pain a "symptom," or is the pain the actual "cause"? Recall what Dr. Ida Rolf, the founder of the Rolfing technique, said: "Where you think the pain is, the problem is not." I truly believe in this statement when I assess my patients.

During the initiation talk with the rowing squad, one of the questions I ask is: "Who has back pain?" The response is generally fairly consistent: around 30–40% of the whole squad say they do, with the percentage being a bit less or a bit more from one year to the next. Of the 30–40%, I can guarantee that in at least 50–60% of these rowers presenting with lower back pain, the Gmax is the main culprit of their perceived symptoms.

If I am honest I can mention numerous specific cases of lower back pain with the main cause being some issue that incorporated the Gmax. For this book, however, I will focus on one case study in particular, involving a patient whom I will call *Mr. Fit*.

Mr. Fit is a 24-year-old elite rower who has competed at Olympic level, so his rowing technique ought to be faultless; this was indeed the case, as the rowing coaches had done their job properly. For as long as Mr. Fit remembers, there had always been an issue with his so-called "tight" hamstrings and painful lower back. The more he was active in rowing, the worse he would feel in relation to his lower back pain and perception of tight hamstrings. He would say to me that he always stretched his hamstrings every day and yet he has never felt any improvement in the length of these muscles, no matter how much stretching he does.

Most rowers will train with weights and often perform bodyweight exercises to help promote the inner core strength and stability required to be an effective team member in whichever discipline of rowing they pursue. This type of training is regularly scheduled in their program and is generally very positive for the progression of the athlete. Nevertheless, in some instances the specific training the rower follows religiously can be detrimental to their overall well-being and can be the precursor of pain later on in their rowing career.

Before becoming an osteopath, I was a physical trainer in the British Army, so I am very experienced in training and implementing the physical requirements of athletes. During my time in the army I have seen numerous injuries that I feel result from incorrect training; the mentality of the forces used to be that when you are told to jump, you reply "How high?" because you do not question what you are told to do. I am pleased to say that things are different today, and now that training programs have advanced over the last 10 years, fewer soldiers and athletes are getting injured.

Exercise History

Through specific questioning in the consultation with Mr. Fit, it became clear that for many years he had been following a heavy weight-training program that focused a lot on deep squatting, dead lifting, and full sit-ups using medicine balls.

Mr. Fit was asked to demonstrate some of the exercises he was doing in his workouts; I asked to see in particular his technique for squats, dead lifts, and lunges. Without going into too much detail, when Mr. Fit performed squats and lunges, his knees were seen to deviate medially on the eccentric motion of the exercise, and the overall movement looked unstable. Because of the athlete's perceived tightness in his hamstrings, his ROM was very limited when demonstrating the dead lift. He was observed to round his lower back rather than keep his lumbar spine in a neutral position, which meant that most of the movement through this exercise was performed using his lower back and hardly any other muscles.

The full sit-ups that Mr. Fit had done every day for as long as he could remember were overactivating his iliopsoas: the iliopsoas is the main prime mover in the full sit-up, so this is not a good abdominal exercise. He had been advised to perform sit-ups to counteract his lower back pain by a physical therapist who had told him that they were "good core exercises," but the exercise was in fact over time causing his iliopsoas to become chronically short and tight. I strongly disagree with the physical therapist's comment that full sit-ups are a good core exercise, and told Mr. Fit that the continual use of this exercise was one of the reasons why his lower back pain was being maintained. From that day onward Mr. Fit stopped doing full sit-ups and began to add in alternative exercises that I showed him.

On Examination

Mr. Fit's posture was very lordotic in the lumbar region, with a bilateral anterior tilt of his pelvis; pain was localized to his central lower back, around the L5/S1 region. The following muscles when tested were found to be in a shortened position and what I would consequently consider to be tight:

- Iliopsoas
- Rectus femoris
- Adductors
- Lumbar erector spinae
- Quadratus lumborum

Figure 5.6 shows that when the specified muscles contract, the innominate will rotate in an anterior direction, which will subsequently cause an anterior tilt and a lumbar lordosis.

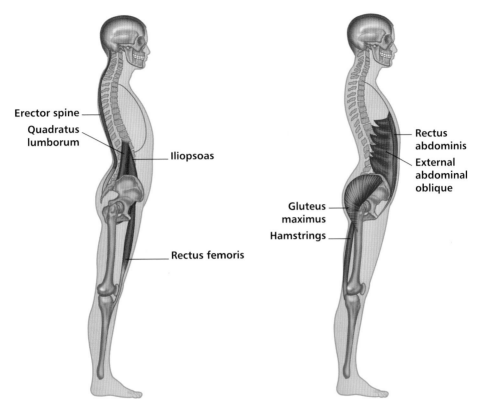

Erector spine
Quadratus
lumborum
Iliopsoas
Rectus femoris

Rectus
abdominis
External
abdominal
oblique
Gluteus
maximus
Hamstrings

Figure 5.6: Hyperlordotic position and the muscles responsible.

Figure 5.7: Muscles responsible for a posterior tilt or a posterior rotation of the innominate.

I will focus more on the muscles in the above list (and in particular the iliopsoas) in chapter 8, as I consider these tight muscle groups to be responsible for a lot of lower back pain. For now, I want to look at what happens to the antagonistic muscles in figure 5.7 when we have this altered posture.

You can see that the posture demonstrated in figure 5.6 exhibits an anterior tilt with a lumbar lordosis; the muscles listed are those responsible for bringing the pelvis back into a neutral position by rotating the innominate posteriorly, as well as causing the lumbar spine to flex. However, because of the increased anterior tilt and lordosis, the muscles that are listed (gluteus muscles, abdominals) are forced into a lengthened position. These muscles can therefore become weak as a compensatory consequence through a neurological inhibition due to the opposite muscles being held in a shortened position (iliopsoas, rectus femoris, and lumbar spine erector spinae).

Gmax Firing Pattern Assessment

Next in my assessment criteria I wanted to evaluate the functional capability of the Gmax of Mr. Fit, as this is the main rowing-stroke muscle that helps to propel the boat effectively. When I performed the hip extension firing pattern test on him (see figure 5.3) he was very much "misfiring on all cylinders"—excuse the expression, but he was. He was so dominant in the hamstrings and the ipsilateral lumbar spine that the Gmax was virtually "asleep" and I felt it was lying very dormant as if it had been switched off.

Treatment

My treatment protocol for Mr. Fit was to follow a plan that is basically outlined in the individual chapters of this book; the treatment and rehabilitation sessions took place at regular intervals and incorporated exercise and remedial therapy as demonstrated and discussed throughout the forthcoming chapters. Indeed, one could say that this entire book has been written on the basis of Mr. Fit's treatment plan, with a focus on this particular case study to give you, the reader, a better understanding of dysfunctional patterns and how we as therapists need to think outside the box in order to properly carry out rehabilitation. (In the case of Mr. Fit, I am pleased to report that my treatment regime successfully resolved his lower back and hamstrings problems, and enabled him to continue with competitive rowing free from these limitations.)

I would like you to read carefully each of the following chapters and then come to your own conclusions about this case study and treatment plan. Give some thought to the differential diagnosis and hypothesis, and to my eventual conclusion and how realistically I had to approach this individual's treatment in order to fix, rather than just relieve, the symptom and underlying problem. Failure to do this might otherwise have led to an exacerbation of symptoms and further problems later on.

Conclusion

As you read each of the following chapters I hope that another piece of the jigsaw puzzle will fall into place, with the final piece being located—and therefore everything becoming apparent—in chapter 12. I am sure that when you read certain sections you will at times doubt, question, or agree with my thought process; by the end, however, I hope you will have a better understanding. Moreover, I hope that I will have given you food for thought so that you start to think about the body as a whole and familiarize yourself with slings and chains and dysfunctional patterns. You will then be able to confidently use various types of therapy and specific exercises to fully rehabilitate your patients/clients. Try to understand my thought process and clinical reasoning in coming to a particular conclusion and in reaching a decision on the course of remedial action that I felt was necessary to take.

The case study outlined above for Mr. Fit is just one example of many possible and diverse situations that can be encountered at a sports injury clinic. Table 5.3 shows, on the left, some common examples of pain and dysfunction that an athlete, or even a non-athletic patient, can present with; the potential findings for their presenting symptoms are shown on the right side of the table.

Athlete presents with	What can it imply?	Likely finding
Tight/painful hamstrings or lumbar paraspinal muscles	Faulty posterior chain muscle activation pattern	Gmax weakness or delayed timing on same side
Insufficient forward or upward power production from the legs		
Pelvic position dropped when running		
Tight/painful adductor magnus (inner thigh) Asymmetrical body orientation	Faulty hip extension pattern: adductor magnus being over used to extend the hip	Gmax function decreased on same side
Asymmetrical body orientation		
Better balance one side than the other		
Excessively tight latissimus dorsi (remembering that the dominant arm will often be slightly less flexible than the non-dominant one)	Faulty posterior oblique sling	Gmax function decreased on opposite side

Table 5.3: Gmax summary. (Source: Elphinston 2013)

Functional Anatomy of the Gluteus Medius

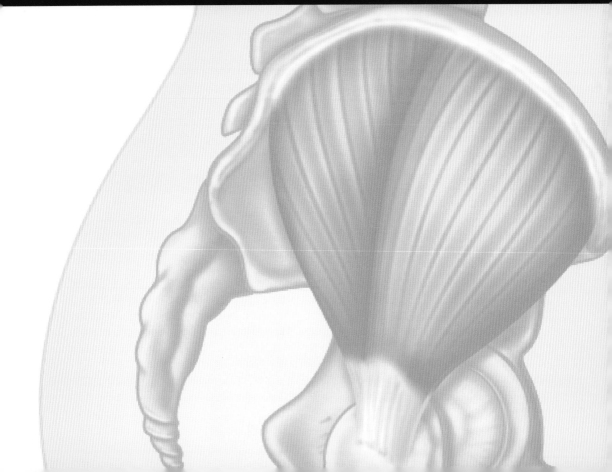

Gmed Anatomy

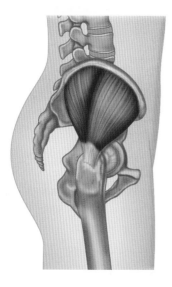

Origin
Outer surface of the ilium, inferior to the iliac crest, between the posterior gluteal line and the anterior gluteal line.

Insertion
Oblique ridge on the lateral surface of the greater trochanter of the femur.

Action
Upper fibers: Laterally rotate and may assist in abduction of the hip joint.
Anterior fibers: Medially rotate and may assist in flexion of the hip joint.
Posterior fibers: Laterally rotate and extend the hip joint.

Nerve
Superior gluteal nerve (L4, L5, S1).

Figure 6.1: Origin, insertion, action, and nerve innervation of the Gmed.

Function of the Gmed

As explained in chapter 3 the Gmed is predominantly used in the gait cycle, especially during the initial contact with the ground and the stance phase of the cycle. Broadly speaking, the Gmed is responsible for maintaining the position of the pelvis as we walk from A to B.

The Gmed should be assessed in every running injury that a patient may present with. Many athletes present to my clinic with overuse running types of injury to the lower limb and trunk, and the majority of them present with poor Gmed function. I have come to the conclusion that the strength and control of this muscle is probably the most important overall component in achieving a biomechanically efficient running pattern. This is not so surprising when you consider that during running you are always either completely in the air or dynamically balanced on one leg. All physical therapist practitioners should be able to assess and restore the Gmed function.

Let's take a closer look at the anatomy of the Gmed: the muscle attaches to the entire length of the iliac crest, to the external ilium between the posterior and anterior gluteal lines, to the gluteal fascia, to the posterior border of the TFL, and to the overlying ITB. The Gmed is divided into three distinct portions—anterior, middle, and posterior—which collectively form a broad conjoined tendon that wraps around, and inserts onto, the greater trochanter of the femur. The more vertical anterior and middle portions of the Gmed appear to be in a better position for abducting the hip than is the more horizontal posterior portion.

There has been much debate over whether the Gmed is primarily activated during medial rotation or during lateral rotation. In 2003 a study by Ireland et al. demonstrated that hip abduction and lateral rotation were significantly weaker in female subjects with patellofemoral pain than in matched controls. This weakness of lateral rotation was attributed to Gmed dysfunction. In contrast, Earl (2005) observed the highest activation of the Gmed in tasks that involved a combination of abduction and medial rotation.

As mentioned above, the Gmed has a posterior fiber in its structure as well as an anterior component; it is the posterior fibers that we as therapists are concerned with. The Gmed posterior fibers work in conjunction with the Gmax, and these muscles control the position of the hip into an external rotation, which helps to align the hip, knee, and lower limb as the gait cycle is initiated.

As an example, consider a patient who is asked to walk while the therapist observes the process. When the patient puts their weight on their *left* leg at the initial contact phase of the cycle, the Gmed is responsible in part for the stability mechanism acting on the lower limb; this will also assist in the overall alignment of the lower limb. The patient continues with the gait cycle and now enters the stance phase. The Gmed in this phase is responsible for abducting the *right* hip, which is then seen to start to lift slightly higher than the *left* side. This process is very important, as it allows the *right* leg to swing during the swing phase of gait.

If there is any weakness in the *left* Gmed, the body will respond in two ways during the gait cycle: either the pelvis will tip down on the contralateral side to the stance leg (*right* in this case), giving the appearance of a Trendelenburg pattern of gait (figure 6.2(a)); or a compensatory Trendelenburg pattern will be adopted, in which the patient will be observed to shift their whole trunk excessively to the weaker hip (figure 6.2(b)).

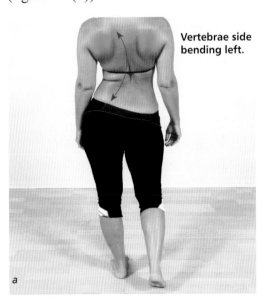
Vertebrae side bending left.

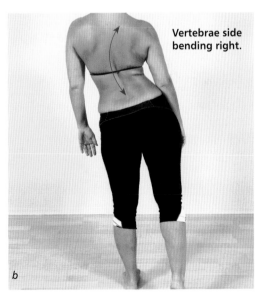
Vertebrae side bending right.

Figure 6.2: (a) Trendelenburg gait; (b) Compensatory Trendelenburg gait.

When we stand on one leg, we activate the lateral sling, which consists of the Gmed, Gmin, adductors on the ipsilateral side, and the QL on the contralateral side (figure 6.3). As explained earlier, if we present with weakness, this is probably a result of overactivation in other muscles owing to the compensation process. Patients who present with weakness in their Gmed (posterior fibers) tend to have overactivity of the adductors and ITB via the connection from the TFL; the piriformis can also have an overactive role if the Gmed posterior fibers are shown to be weak.

The Gmed is key to dynamic pelvic stability. In my experience, runners with poor dynamic pelvic stability will shorten their stride length and adopt a more shuffling pattern to reduce the ground reaction force at contact and thereby decrease the amount of muscle control required to maintain pelvic posture.

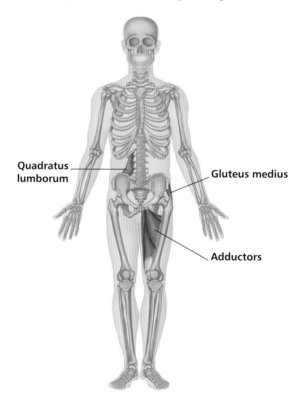

Figure 6.3: Lateral sling.

Gmed weakness will have implications all the way down the kinetic chain. From heel contact to the mid-stance phase, a weakness of the Gmed allows:

- excessive adduction and internal rotation of the femur;
- the knee to drift into a valgus or possibly varus position;
- the lower limb (tibia) to rotate internally relative to the position of the foot;
- increased weight transfer to the medial aspect of the foot;
- increased pronation of the STJ.

As you can see from the above consequences of a weakness in the function of the Gmed, the athlete is at continual risk of any sports-related injury condition relating to increased and/or prolonged over-pronation of the STJ, such as medial tibial stress syndrome (shin splints), plantar fasciitis, or Achilles tendinopathy.

A strong Gmax and Gmed is a stable knee.

Assessment of the Gmed

Whenever I look at patients who present with knee or lower lumbar spine pain, part of my assessment process includes checking the strength of the gluteal muscles and in particular the Gmed. In this section I will discuss the hip abduction firing pattern test, which is used for determining the correct firing order of the hip abductors (including the Gmed muscle).

Hip Abduction Firing Pattern Test

To check the firing sequence on the left side, the patient adopts a side-lying posture with both legs together and their left leg on top. In this sequence, three muscles will be tested: Gmed, TFL, and QL. The therapist palpates the QL muscle by placing their right hand lightly on the muscle. Next, to palpate the Gmed and TFL, the therapist placed their finger on the TFL and their thumb on the Gmed, as shown in figures 6.4(a) and (b).

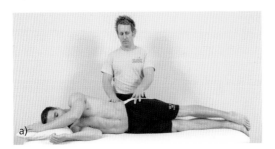 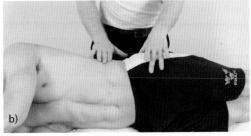

Figure 6.4: (a) Palpation of the QL, Gmed, and TFL; (b) Close-up of the hand position.

The patient is asked to lift their left leg into abduction, a few inches from their right leg, while the therapist notes the firing sequence (figure 6.5). It is important to check for any compensatory or cheating recruitment. The idea of this test is that the patient must be able to abduct their hip without (1) hitching the left side of their pelvis (hip hitching would mean they were activating the quadratus lumborum), (2) falling into an anterior pelvic tilt, or (3) allowing their pelvis to tip backward.

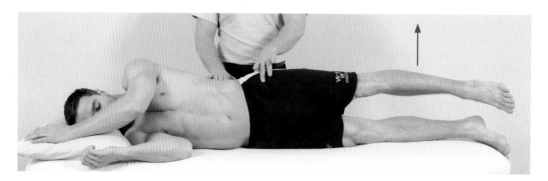

Figure 6.5: As the patient abducts their left hip, the therapist notes the firing sequence.

The correct firing sequence should be Gmed, followed by TFL, and finally QL at around 25 degrees of pelvis elevation. If the QL or the TFL fires first, this indicates a misfiring sequence, resulting in adaptive shortness.

Once we have ascertained the firing sequence for hip abduction, we have to decide on the next step. Most patients feel that they need to strengthen the weak Gmed muscle by going to the gym, especially if they have been told it is weak, and they do lots of side-lying abduction exercises. The difficulty in strengthening the apparent weak Gmed muscle is that this particular exercise will not, I repeat *not*, strengthen the Gmed, especially if the TFL and QL are the dominant abductors. The piriformis will also get involved, as it is a weak abductor, which can cause a pelvic/sacroiliac dysfunction, further complicating the underlying issue.

So the answer is to initially postpone the strengthening of the Gmed and focus on the shortened/tight tissues of the adductors, TFL, and QL. In theory, by lengthening the tight tissues, the lengthened and weakened tissue will become shorter and automatically regain its strength. If, after a period of time (two weeks has been recommended), the Gmed has not regained its strength, specific and functional strength exercises for this muscle can be added.

Gluteus Medius Anterior/Posterior Fibers Strength Test

To test the left Gmed, the patient adopts a side-lying posture, with their left leg uppermost. The therapist palpates the patient's Gmed with their right hand, and the patient is asked to raise their left leg into abduction, a few inches away from the right leg, and hold this position isometrically to start with. Placing their left hand near the patient's knee, the therapist applies a downward pressure to the leg. The patient is asked to resist the pressure (figure 6.6); if they are able to do so, the Gmed is classified as *normal*.

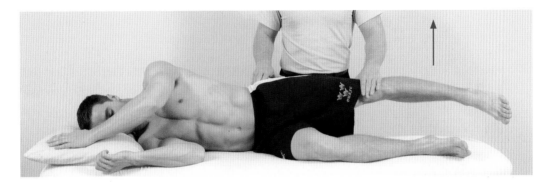

Figure 6.6: The patient abducting their left hip against resistance from the therapist.

Gluteus Medius Posterior Fibers Strength Test

In testing the left side, to put more emphasis on the posterior fibers of the Gmed, the therapist controls the patient's left hip into slight extension and external rotation, as shown in figure 6.7. The therapist applies a downward pressure as before (figure 6.8); if the patient is able to resist this force, the Gmed posterior fibers are classified as *normal*. If you want to assess muscular endurance as opposed to strength, ask the patient to hold the abducted leg and maintain the position for at least 30 seconds.

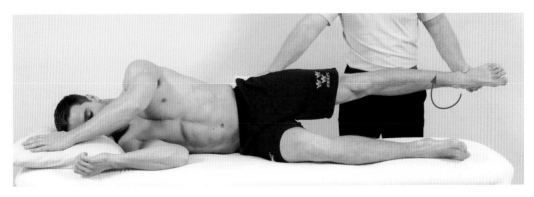

Figure 6.7: External rotation of the hip, which emphasizes the posterior fibers of the Gmed.

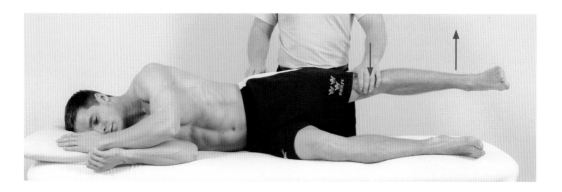

Figure 6.8: The therapist applies a downward pressure to the patient's abducted hip.

The information presented in table 6.1 (similar to table 5.3 in chapter 5 for the Gmax) will enable you to identify possible pain and dysfunctions that are related to the Gmed.

Athlete presents with	What can it imply?	Likely finding
Swagger or pendulum gait	Faulty weight bearing strategy	Gmed weakness/timing problem
Tight quadratus lumborum (side trunk muscles)	Difficulty orientating the trunk vertically over the pelvis in gait, requiring overuse of side trunk muscles	Gmed dysfunction either side
Tight piriformis	Faulty pelvic control in weight bearing requiring greater coronal plane control	Gmed dysfunction same side
Tight ITB/lateral knee pain/knee cap pain	Faulty hip abduction or hip flexion strategy	Dysfunction of Gmed or psoas, same side

Table 6.1: Gmed summary. (Source: Elphinston 2013)

Muscle Energy Techniques

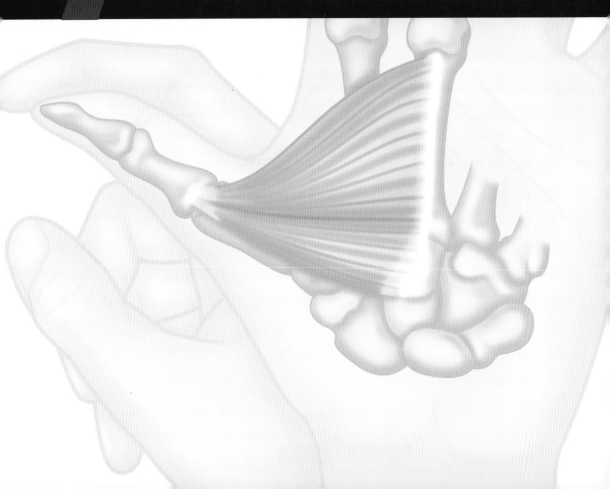

Since I am discussing how to maximize the glutes through lengthening the tight antagonist muscles, I need to explain the role of muscle energy techniques (METs) so that you have a better understanding of when and why to employ this type of treatment. Physical therapists have a toolbox of various techniques at their disposal to help release and relax muscles, which will then assist the patient's body to promote the healing mechanisms. METs, first described by Mitchell in 1948, are one such tool that if used correctly can have a major influence on the patient's well-being. (The reader is referred to Gibbons (2012) for a fuller account of METs.)

> **Definition:** *Muscle energy techniques (METs)* are a form of osteopathic manipulative diagnosis and treatment in which the patient's muscles are actively used on request, from a precisely controlled position, in a specific direction, and against a distinctly executed counterforce.

METs are unique in their application in that the patient provides the initial effort and the practitioner just facilitates the process. The primary force comes from the contraction of the patient's soft tissues (muscles), which is then utilized to assist and correct the presenting musculoskeletal dysfunction. This treatment method is generally classified as a *direct* form of technique as opposed to *indirect*, since the use of muscular effort is from a controlled position, in a specific direction, and against a distant counterforce that is usually offered by the practitioner.

Some of the Benefits of METs

When teaching the concept of METs to my students, one of the benefits I emphasize is their use in normalizing joint range, rather than in improving flexibility. This might sound counterintuitive; what I am saying is if, for example, your patient cannot rotate their neck (cervical spine) to the right as far as they can to the left, they have a restriction of the cervical spine in a right rotation. The normal rotational range of the cervical spine is 80 degrees, but let's say the patient can only rotate 70 degrees to the right. This is where METs come in. After an MET has been employed on the tight restrictive muscles, hopefully the cervical spine will then be capable of rotating to 80 degrees—the patient has made all the effort and you, the practitioner, have encouraged the cervical spine into further right rotation. You have now improved the joint range to "normal." This is not stretching in the strictest sense—even though the overall flexibility has been improved, it is only to the point of achieving what is considered to be a normal joint range.

Depending on the context and the type of MET employed, the objectives of this treatment can include:

- Restoring normal tone in hypertonic muscles
- Strengthening weak muscles
- Preparing muscles for subsequent stretching
- Increasing joint mobility

Restoring Normal Tone in Hypertonic Muscles

Through the simple process of METs, we as physical therapists try to achieve a relaxation in the hypertonic shortened muscles. If we think of a joint as being limited in its ROM, then through the initial identification of the hypertonic structures, we can employ the techniques to help achieve normality in the tissues. Certain types of massage therapy can also help us achieve this relaxation effect, and generally an MET is applied in conjunction with massage therapy. I personally feel that massage with motion is one of the best tools a physical therapist has.

Strengthening Weak Muscles

METs can be used in the strengthening of weak or even flaccid muscles, as the patients are asked to contract the muscles prior to the lengthening process. The therapist should be able to modify the MET by asking the patient to contract the muscle that has been classified as *weak*, against a resistance applied by the therapist (isometric contraction), the timing of which can be varied. For example, the patient can be asked to resist the movement using approximately 20–30% of their maximum capability for 5–15 seconds. They are then asked to repeat the process five to eight times, resting for 10–15 seconds between repetitions. The patient's performance can be noted and improved over time.

Preparing Muscles for Subsequent Stretching

In certain circumstances, what sport your patient participates in will be determined by what ROM they have at their joints. Everybody can improve their flexibility, and METs can be used to help achieve this goal. Remember that the focus of METs is to try to improve the normal ROM of a joint.

If you want to improve the patient's flexibility past the point of normal, a more aggressive MET approach might be recommended. This could be in the form of asking the patient to contract a bit firmer than the standard 10–20% of the muscle's capability. For example, we can ask the patient to contract using, say, 40–70% of the muscle's capability. This increased contraction will help stimulate more motor units to fire, in turn causing an increased stimulation of the Golgi tendon organ (GTO). This will then have the effect of relaxing more of the muscle, allowing it to be lengthened even further. Either way, once an MET has been incorporated into the treatment plan, a flexibility program can follow.

Increasing Joint Mobility

One of my favorite sayings when I teach muscle testing courses is: "A stiff joint can become a tight muscle, and a tight muscle can become a stiff joint." Does this not make perfect sense?

When you use an MET correctly, it is one of the best ways to improve the mobility of the joint, even though you are relaxing the muscles initially. The focus of the MET is to get the patient to contract the muscles; this subsequently causes a relaxation period, allowing a greater ROM to be achieved within that specific joint.

Physiological Effects of METs

Postural deviations are described in chapter 2 and by using the techniques demonstrated in this book, we can initially identify which muscles are classified as *short* and what effects this has on one's body position and the relationship to the glutes. Once these muscles have been identified through the given specific tests, we will be able to use an MET to help correct these dysfunctions; a corrective treatment plan can then be designed to help maximize the glutes.

There are two main effects of METs and these are explained on the basis of two distinct physiological processes:

- Post-isometric relaxation (PIR)
- Reciprocal inhibition (RI)

When we use METs, certain neurological influences occur. Before we discuss the main process of PIR/RI, we need to consider the two types of receptor involved in the stretch reflex:

- Muscle spindles, which are sensitive to change, and speed of change, in length of muscle fibers
- GTOs, which detect prolonged change in tension

Stretching the muscle causes an increase in the impulses transmitted from the muscle spindle to the posterior horn cell (PHC) of the spinal cord. In turn, the anterior horn cell (AHC) transmits an increase in motor impulses to the muscle fibers, creating a protective tension to resist the stretch. However, increased tension after a few seconds is sensed within the GTOs, which transmit impulses to the PHC. These impulses have an inhibitory effect on the increased motor stimulus at the AHC. This inhibitory effect causes a reduction in motor impulses and consequent relaxation. This implies that the prolonged stretch of the muscles will increase the stretching capability because the protective relaxation of the GTOs overrides the protective contraction due to the muscle spindles. A fast stretch of the muscle spindles, however, will cause immediate muscle contraction and since it is not sustained, there will be no inhibitory action. This is known as the *basic reflex arc*.

PIR results from a neurological feedback through the spinal cord to the muscle itself when an isometric contraction is sustained, causing a reduction in tone of the muscle which has been contracted. This reduction in tone lasts for approximately 20–25 seconds, during which time the tissues can be more easily moved to a new resting length.

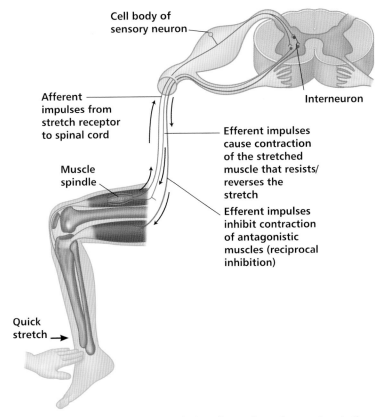

Figure 7.1: The 'stretch reflex arc'. A quick 'stretch by hand' to activate the muscle spindles.

When RI is employed, the reduction in tone relies on the physiological inhibiting effect of antagonists on the contraction of a muscle. When the motor neurons of the contracting agonist muscle receive excitatory impulses from the afferent pathway, the motor neurons of the opposing antagonist muscle receive inhibitory impulses at the same time, which prevent it contracting. It follows that contraction or extended stretch of the agonist muscle must elicit relaxation or inhibit the antagonist; however, a fast stretch of the agonist will facilitate a contraction of the agonist.

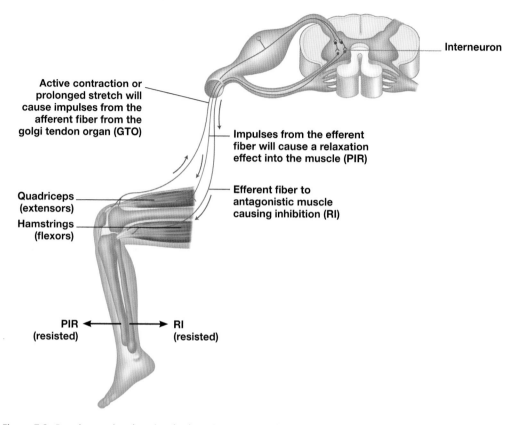

Figure 7.2: Post-isometric relaxation (PIR), and reciprocal inhibition (RI).

A refractory period (the brief period needed to restore the resting potential) of about 20 seconds occurs with RI; however, RI is thought to be less powerful than PIR. Therapists need to be able to use both approaches, because the use of the agonist may sometimes be inappropriate owing to pain or injury. Since the amount of force used with an MET is minimal, the risk of injury or tissue damage will be reduced.

MET Method of Application

"Point of Bind" or the "Restriction Barrier"

In this book the word "bind" is mentioned numerous times. The *point of bind*, or *restriction barrier*, occurs when resistance is first felt by the palpating hand/fingers of the therapist. Through experience and continual practice, the therapist will be able to palpate a resistance of the soft tissues as the affected area is gently taken into the position of bind. This position of bind is not the position of stretch—it is the position just before the point of stretch. The therapist should be able to feel the difference and not wait for the patient to say when they feel a stretch has occurred.

In most applications of METs, the point of bind, or just short of the point of bind, is the preferred position in which to perform an MET. Clearly, an MET is a fairly mild form of stretching compared with other techniques, so one can assume it is therefore more appropriate in the rehabilitation process. It should be borne in mind that most problems with muscle shortening will occur in postural muscles. Since these muscles are composed predominantly of slow-twitch fibers, a milder form of stretching is perhaps more appropriate.

Procedure

- The patient's limb is taken to the point where resistance is felt, i.e. the point of bind. It can be more comfortable for the patient if you ease off to a point slightly short of the point of bind in the affected area that you are going to treat, especially if these tissues are in the chronic stage.
- The patient is asked to isometrically contract the muscle to be treated (PIR) or the antagonist (RI), using approximately 10–20% of the muscle's strength capability against a resistance that is applied by the therapist.
- The patient should be using the agonist if the method of approach is PIR; this will release the tight, shortened structures directly.
- If the RI method of MET is used, the patient is asked to contract the antagonist isometrically; this will induce a relaxation effect in the opposite muscle group (agonist) that would still be classified as the *tight* and *shortened* structures. (See the PIR example below.)
- The patient is asked to slowly introduce an isometric contraction, lasting between 10 and 12 seconds, avoiding any jerking of the treated area. This contraction, as explained above, is the time necessary to load the GTOs, which allows them to become active and to influence the intrafusal fibers from the muscle spindles. This has the effect of overriding the influence from the muscle spindles, which inhibits muscle tone. The therapist then has the opportunity to take the affected area to a new position with minimal effort.
- The contraction by the patient should cause no discomfort or strain.
- The patient is told to relax fully by taking a deep breath in, and as they breathe out, the therapist passively takes the specific joint that lengthens the hypertonic muscle to a new position, which therefore normalizes joint range.
- After an isometric contraction, which induces a PIR, there is a relaxation period of 15–30 seconds; this period can be the perfect time to stretch the tissues to their new resting length.
- Repeat this process until no further progress is made (normally three to four times) and hold the final resting position for approximately 25–30 seconds. A period of 25–30 seconds is considered to be enough time for the neurological system to lock onto this new resting position.
- This type of technique is excellent for relaxing and releasing tone in tight, shortened soft tissues.

Acute and Chronic Conditions

The soft tissue conditions that are treated using METs are generally classified as either *acute* or *chronic*, and this tends to relate to tissues that have had some form of strain or trauma. METs can be used for both acute and chronic conditions. Acute involves anything that is obviously acute in terms of symptoms, pain, or spasm, as well as anything that has emerged during the previous three to four weeks. Anything older and of a less obviously acute nature is regarded as chronic in determining which variation of MET is suitable.

If you feel the presenting condition is relatively acute (occurring within the last three weeks), the isometric contraction can be performed at the point of bind. After the patient has contracted the muscle isometrically for the duration of 10 seconds, the therapist then takes the affected area to the new point of bind.

In chronic conditions (persisting for more than three weeks), the isometric contraction starts from a position just before the point of bind. After the patient has contracted the muscle for 10 seconds, the therapist then goes through the point of bind and encourages the specific area into the new position.

PIR versus RI

How much pain the patient is presenting with is generally the deciding factor in determining which method to initially apply. The PIR method is usually the technique of choice for muscles that are classified as *short* and *tight*, as it is these muscles that are initially contracted in the process of releasing and relaxing.

However, on occasion the patient experiences discomfort when the agonist, i.e. the shortened structure, is contracted; in this case it would seem more appropriate to contract the opposite muscle group (antagonist), as this would reduce the patient's perception of pain, but still induce a relaxation in the painful tissues. Hence, the use of the RI method, using the antagonists, which are usually pain free, will generally be the first choice if there is increased sensitivity in the primary shortened tissues.

When the patient's initial pain has been reduced by the appropriate treatment, PIR techniques can be incorporated (as explained earlier, PIR uses an isometric contraction of the tight shortened structures, in contrast to the antagonists being used in the RI method). To some extent, the main factor in deciding the best approach is whether the sensitive tissue is in the acute stage or in the chronic stage.

After having used PIR and RI on a regular basis, I have found that the best results of lengthening the hypertonic structures are achieved with PIR (provided the patient has no pain during this technique). However, once I have performed the PIR method, if I feel more ROM is needed in the shortened tight tissue, I bring into play the antagonists using the RI method for approximately two more repetitions. This approach for my patients has had the desired effect of improving the overall ROM.

PIR Example

We are now going to apply a PIR method of MET treatment to the adductor pollicis muscle (*pollicis* relates to the thumb, or pollex). You might consider it more appropriate to demonstrate how METs work by means of an example related the glutes; however, I wanted the therapist to be able to practice the technique on themselves first, so that they can better understand the MET concept. Once the technique has been understood and subsequently practiced using this simple example, the therapist will then be ready to tackle more complex METs with the aim of helping to restore function to the vital glutes.

Place your left (or right) hand onto a blank piece of paper and, with the hand open as much as possible, draw around the fingers and the thumb (figure 7.3).

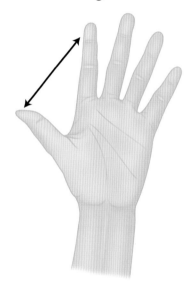

Figure 7.3: The distance between the thumb and finger is measured.

Remove the paper and actively abduct the thumb as far as you can, until a point of bind is felt. Next, place the fingers of your right hand on top of the left thumb and, using an isometric contraction, adduct your thumb against the downward pressure of the fingers, so that an isometric contraction is achieved (figure 7.4). After applying this pressure for 10 seconds, breathe in, and on the exhalation passively take the thumb into further abduction (but do not force the thumb). Repeat this sequence two more times and on the last repetition, hold the isometric contraction for at least 20–25 seconds.

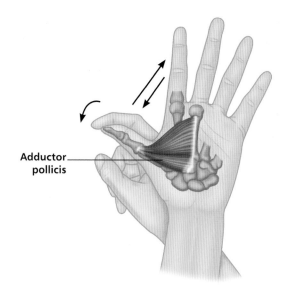

Figure 7.4: Adducting the thumb against a resistance applied by the opposite hand.

Now place your hand back on the piece of paper and draw around it again (figure 7.5); hopefully you will see that the thumb has abducted further than before.

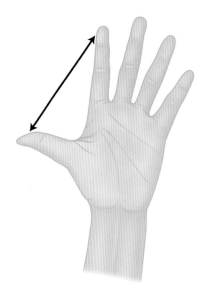

Figure 7.5: The hand redrawn after the MET treatment using PIR.

The Antagonistic Cause—the Vital Iliopsoas, Rectus Femoris, and Adductors

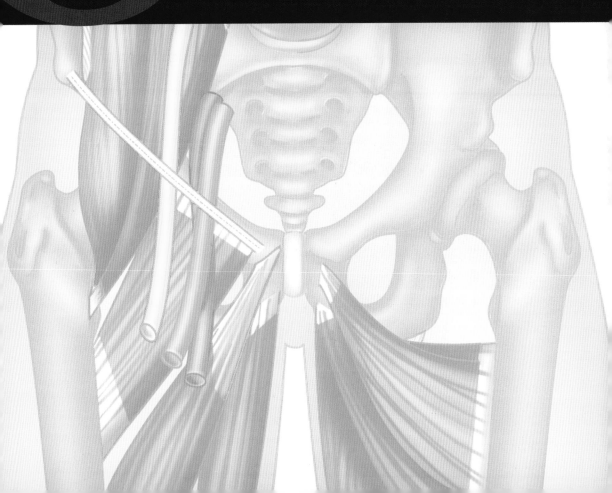

The focus of this chapter will be to identify the relative shortness and subsequent tightness patterns within soft tissue structures, i.e. specific muscles that are prone to shortening and becoming tight. I have already discussed why the antagonistic muscles can become lengthened and weakened; this is applicable to both the Gmax and the Gmed, as they are both part of the phasic muscle group. The remedy is not to strengthen the so-called "weak" muscles: encouraging strength-based exercise will not assist these specific muscles in regaining their muscular strength, since they are held in a weakened position by the short and tight antagonists.

Sherrington's law of reciprocal inhibition (Sherrington 1907) states that a hypertonic antagonist muscle may be reflexively inhibiting its agonist. Therefore, in the presence of short and subsequently tight antagonistic muscles, we must first look at restoring normal muscle tone and/or length before attempting to strengthen a weakened or inhibited muscle. The answer is to somehow change the hypertonicity of these shortened muscles by encouraging them to lengthen; this can be done by using a combination of METs (e.g. PIR) and specific myofascial release techniques, before we add in specific strengthening exercises for the glutes as described in chapter 12.

Kankaanpaa et al. (1998) and O'Sullivan et al. (1997) researched the effects of pain inhibition and altered control of lumbopelvic posture on the creation of imbalances in the activation patterns of global muscles such as the Gmax and Gmed. Hungerford et al. (2003) reported that as a result of such imbalances, these muscles may be more actively substituted by the biceps femoris, iliopsoas, TFL, and adductor muscles.

Remember which muscles are antagonistic to the glutes? Well, the Gmax in particular is a powerful hip extensor so its antagonist has to be the hip flexors—the main muscles responsible for hip flexion—specifically the iliopsoas and rectus femoris. The Gmed is a powerful hip abductor so its antagonist has to be the adductors. One way of encouraging a correct hip extension firing pattern is to identify and correct a hip flexor length issue: if the flexors are tested as short, an MET or a myofascial release technique can be utilized to normalize the resting length of these shortened structures. This process of lengthening the shortened structures can be applied for a period of approximately two weeks; if the specific firing pattern has not improved after this time, strengthening protocols for the Gmax can then be incorporated into the treatment plan as described later.

The antagonists of the Gmax and Gmed are therefore:

- Iliopsoas (comprising the psoas major and iliacus)
- Rectus femoris
- Adductors

These muscles will now be discussed in more detail. (There are other associated muscles, but they will not be covered in this book.)

Iliopsoas Anatomy

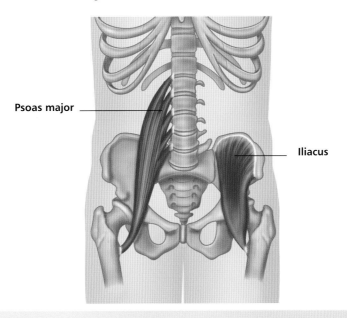

Psoas major

Iliacus

Origin
Psoas major: Transverse processes of all the lumbar vertebrae (L1–L5). Bodies of the 12th thoracic and all lumbar vertebrae (T12–L5). Intervertebral discs above each lumbar vertebra.
Iliacus: Superior two-thirds of the iliac fossa. Anterior ligaments of the lumbosacral and SIJs.

Insertion
Lesser trochanter of the femur.

Action
Main flexor of the hip joint and assists in lateral rotation of the hip. Acting from its insertion, it flexes the trunk, as in sitting up from the supine position.

Nerve
Psoas major: Ventral rami of lumbar nerves (L1–L4).
Iliacus: Femoral nerve (L1– L4).

Figure 8.1: Origin, insertion, action, and nerve innervation of the iliopsoas.

Assessment of the Iliopsoas

Modified Thomas Test

To test the right hip, the patient is asked to lie back on the edge of a couch while holding onto their left knee. As they roll backward, the patient pulls their left knee as far as they can toward their chest, as shown in figure 8.2. The full flexion of the hip encourages full posterior rotation of the innominate bone and helps to flatten the lordosis. From this position, the therapist looks at where the patient's right knee lies, relative to the right hip. The position of the knee should be just below the level of the hip; figure 8.2 demonstrates a normal length of the right iliopsoas.

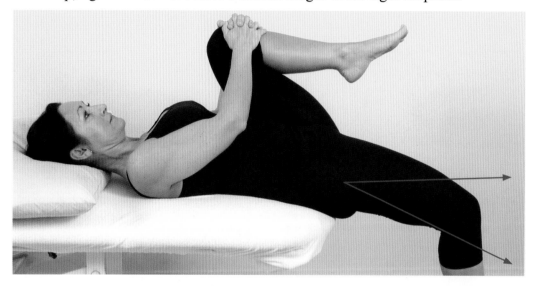

Figure 8.2: The right knee is below the level of the hip, indicating a normal length of the iliopsoas.

In figure 8.3 the therapist is demonstrating with their arms the position of the right hip compared with the right knee. You can see that the hip is held in a flexed position, which confirms the tightness of the right iliopsoas in this case.

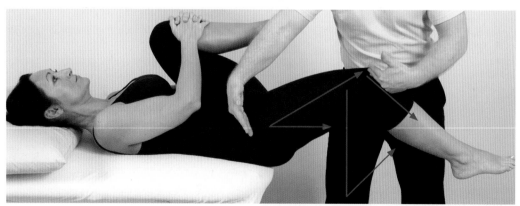

Figure 8.3: A tight right iliopsoas is confirmed. A tight rectus femoris can also be seen.

With the patient in the Modified Thomas Test position, the therapist can apply an abduction of the hip (figure 8.4), and an adduction of the hip (figure 8.5). A range of motion (ROM) of 10–15 degrees for each of these is commonly accepted to be normal.

If the hip is restricted in abduction, i.e. a bind occurs at an angle of less than 10–15 degrees, the muscles of the adductor group are held in a shortened position; if the adduction movement is restricted, the ITB and TFL are held in a shortened position.

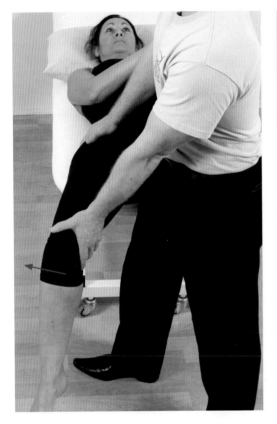 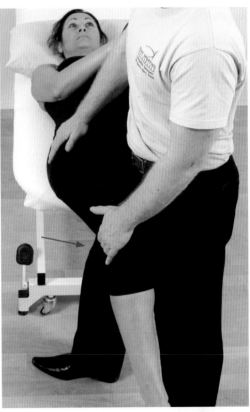

Figure 8.4: Restricted hip abduction, indicating tight adductors.

Figure 8.5: Restricted hip adduction, indicating a tight ITB/TFL.

MET Treatment of the Iliopsoas

To treat the right side, the patient adopts the same position as in the Modified Thomas Test above. The patient's left foot is placed into the therapist's right side and pressure is applied by the therapist to induce full flexion of the patient's left hip. Stabilizing the patient's right hip with their right hand, the therapist puts their left hand just above the patient's right knee. The patient is asked to flex their right hip against the therapist's resistance for 10 seconds, as shown in figure 8.6.

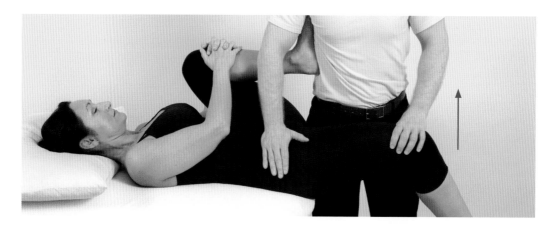

Figure 8.6: The patient flexes their right hip against resistance from the therapist's left hand, while the hip is being stabilized by the therapist's right hand.

Following the isometric contraction, and on the relaxation phase, the therapist slowly applies a downward pressure. This will cause the hip to passively go into extension and will induce a lengthening of the right iliopsoas, as shown in figure 8.7. Gravity will also play a part in this technique, by assisting in the lengthening of the iliopsoas.

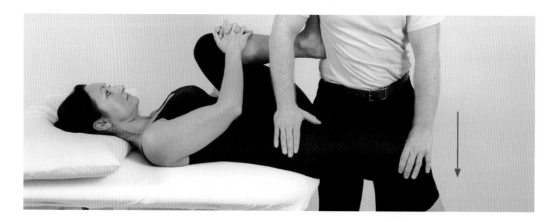

Figure 8.7: The therapist passively extends the hip to lengthen the iliopsoas, with the assistance of gravity.

Alternatively, it is possible to contract the iliopsoas from the flexed position, as shown in figure 8.8. This is normally used if the original method of activating the iliopsoas causes discomfort to the patient. Allowing the hip to be in a more flexed position will slacken the iliopsoas, which will assist in its contraction and help reduce the discomfort.

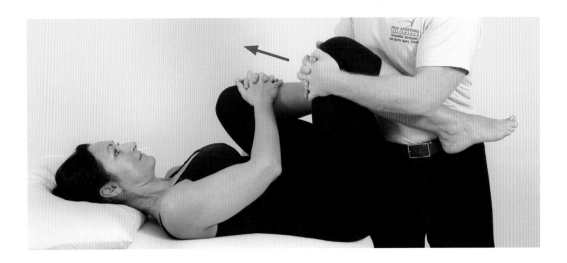

Figure 8.8: The patient resists hip flexion from a flexed position.

The patient is asked to flex their right hip against a resistance applied by the therapist's left hand (figure 8.8). After a 10-second contraction, and on the relaxation phase, the therapist lengthens the iliopsoas by taking the hip into an extended position, as demonstrated in figure 8.9.

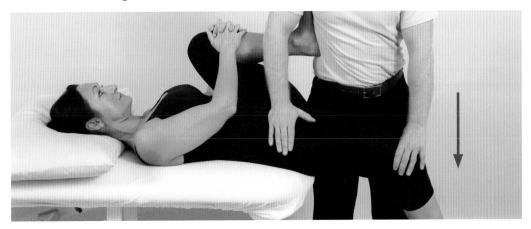

Figure 8.9: Lengthening of the right iliopsoas.

Tip: The psoas major is also known as *filet mignon*, which is a piece of beef taken from the tenderloin. A bilateral shortness of the psoas major can cause the pelvis to anteriorly tilt, in turn causing the lumbar spine to adopt a position of hyperlordosis. This can result in compression of the facet joints, leading to lower back pain.

Note: If full sit-ups are performed on a regular basis, the iliopsoas is predominantly the muscle being used. Repeated sit-ups will make the iliopsoas stronger and tighter, and result in weakness of the abdominals; this can maintain a patient's lower back pain.

To prove the involvement of the iliopsoas, have your patient lie on their back with their knees bent. Hold the patient's ankles and ask them to dorsiflex their ankles while you resist the movement. This will stimulate the anterior chain musculature, including the iliopsoas, which is part of this chain. The patient then performs the full sit-up movement (most fit individuals will be able to do many sit-ups).

To deactivate or switch off the iliopsoas, the patient is asked to plantar flex their ankles (instead of dorsiflexing them), or to squeeze their glutes. Either of these actions stimulates the posterior chain musculature, causing the iliopsoas to switch off, as activation of the gluteal muscles results in a relaxation of the iliopsoas through RI. When the patient is now asked to perform the sit-up, the movement will prove to be impossible, confirming that the iliopsoas is generally the prime mover in a full sit-up.

Myofascial Treatment of the Psoas Major

The psoas major can be involved in numerous patterns of dysfunction generally involving the pelvis and the lumbar and thoracic spines. Some authors suggest that the lower medial fibers can contribute to maintaining a hyperlordotic curve, whereas the upper lateral fibers can contribute to maintaining a flat-back position.

The technique I describe for the release of the psoas major can be very awkward to perform correctly because of the anatomy of the muscle and associated structures of the internal organs. What I am trying to say is that you have to be very careful when attempting to palpate and treat the psoas major as it can and will be very tender, especially if it is held in a shortened position. The physical therapist needs to be guided by an experienced therapist when treating this area and should not try to treat the psoas major just by reading this book.

Locating the Psoas Major

Have your patient supine with their left knee bent and the foot flat. Next locate the umbilicus of the patient and come approximately 2" laterally and 2" caudally (downward), as shown in figure 8.10. This particular area enables the physical therapist to palpate and treat the psoas major. Have the patient bend their knee as before, as this will help relax the psoas major. Start by slowly and gently placing your fingertips through the soft tissues until you make contact with a firmer structure, as shown in figure 8.11. When you feel that you have located the psoas major, ask your patient to lift that leg off the couch an inch and you will feel the contraction of the muscle, which will confirm that you are in the correct area (figure 8.12). If you do not feel the muscle contact, you may need to move a little more medially, toward the spine. Once you are in contact, the patient may report being unable to lift the leg; this might be an indication of a weakened muscle and that the pressure you are applying is causing an inhibition.

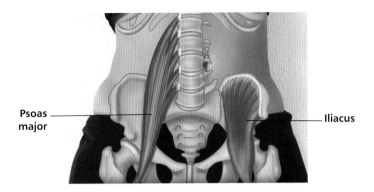

Figure 8.10: Psoas major location as drawn on the abdomen.

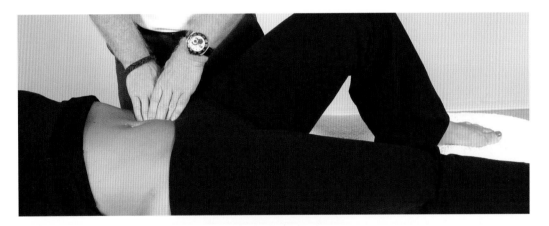

Figure 8.11: Palpation of the left psoas major through the abdomen.

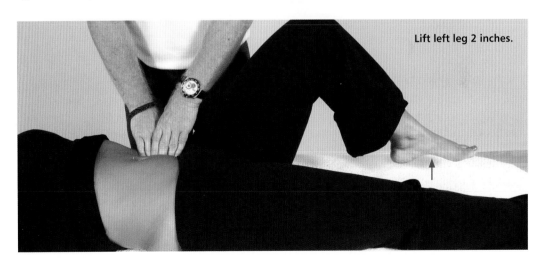

Figure 8.12: Palpation of the left psoas major through the abdomen—left leg lifted.

Start Position
The patient lies supine, with their knees bent. The therapist palpates the left psoas major as explained above, with reinforcement from the fingers of the other hand. The patient is then asked to flex the hip to ascertain the correct positioning of the hands and to isolate the psoas major, as seen in figure 8.12. The lateral fibers of the psoas major are the ones you are most likely to engage. If you want to target the medial fibers, keep in contact with the bulk of the muscle as you slowly roll over it to engage the lower fibers. This will also guide you and help move any fragile structures and vessels out the way before you apply firmer pressure. The patient is then instructed to slide their heel along the couch as slowly as they can while the therapist maintains pressure on the psoas major; this technique is described as "locking" the psoas major as the patient lengthens the muscle (see figure 8.13).

If this concept is difficult to understand, another way of thinking about it is as follows. Imagine inserting a key into a door; this is analogous to your fingers (key) pressing onto the psoas major (door); the patient straightening their leg corresponds to "opening the door."

Once the patient has straightened their leg as far as they can, the therapist eases off on the contact pressure being applied the psoas major, and the procedure is repeated another two or three times, or until a change in the tissue texture is felt.

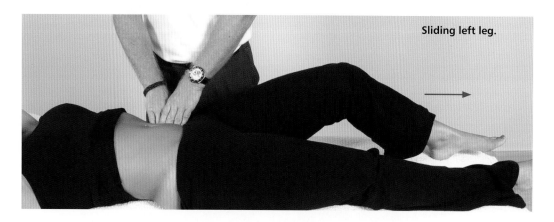

Sliding left leg.

Figure 8.13: Patient lengthens their left leg while the therapist applies pressure to the left psoas major.

Correct breathing technique could also be very beneficial to the lengthening of the psoas major because of the muscle's attachment to the diaphragm. I normally instruct my patient to take a breath in as I apply pressure to the psoas major with my fingertips; as the patient straightens their leg, I ask them to exhale fully on the relaxation phase.

Variations of the Technique
The technique described above is what I call the *starting technique*, as once this is performed correctly, the technique can be slightly altered to achieve a more desirable effect.

As mentioned above, the starting technique is performed by the therapist applying pressure to "lock" the tissue; however, since the therapist's fingertips are in a locked position, a slight pressure can be applied toward the lumbar spine (psoas major origin) as the patient lowers their leg. This might have the effect of encouraging a better lengthening of the psoas major.

Another great technique that I include for lengthening the psoas major, which works very well for me in my clinic, is the use of the arm. The starting position of this technique variation is shown in figure 8.14: the therapist palpates the left psoas major as the patient lifts their left leg 2" off the couch, while lifting their left arm off the couch at the same time. The patient is then asked to breathe in and start straightening their left leg; while exhaling, the patient is instructed to stretch their arm above their head to try to reach as far as is comfortable, as shown in figure 8.15. This procedure seems to have a tremendous effect on lengthening the psoas major.

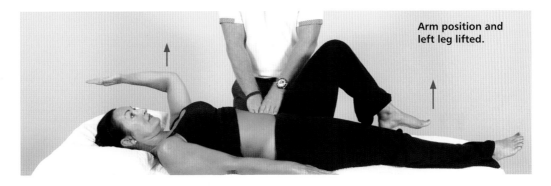

Figure 8.14: Patient in the starting position, with the therapist applying pressure to the left psoas major.

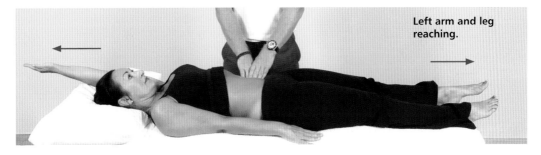

Figure 8.15: Patient straightens their left leg and arm, while the therapist applies pressure to the left psoas major.

A variation of the above technique using the arm is to ask the patient to side bend to the right at the end of the lengthening phase, as shown in figure 8.16.

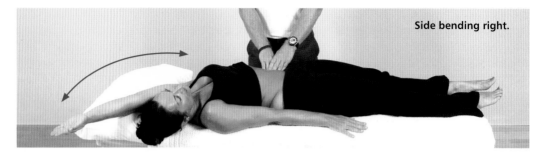

Side bending right.

Figure 8.16: Patient lengthens their left leg and arm and then side bends to the right, while the therapist applies pressure to the left psoas major.

Rectus Femoris Anatomy

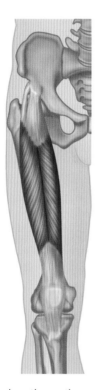

Origin
Straight head (anterior head): Anterior inferior iliac spine.
Reflected head (posterior head): Groove above the acetabulum (on the ilium).

Insertion
Patella, then via the patellar ligament to the tuberosity of the tibia.

Action
Extends the knee joint and flexes the hip joint (particularly in combination movements, such as in kicking a ball). Assists iliopsoas in flexing the trunk on the thigh. Prevents flexion at the knee joint as the heel strikes the ground during walking.

Nerve
Femoral nerve (L2–L4).

Figure 8.17: Origin, insertion, action, and nerve innervation of the rectus femoris.

Assessment of the Rectus Femoris

Modified Thomas Test

This test is an excellent way of identifying shortness not only in the rectus femoris but also in the iliopsoas as explained earlier. To test the right rectus femoris, the patient adopts the position as demonstrated in figure 8.18, in which they are holding onto their left leg.

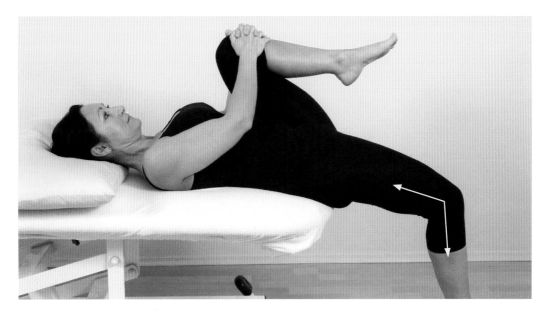

Figure 8.18: To test the right rectus femoris, the patient lies on the couch and holds onto their left leg. A normal length of the rectus femoris is shown.

The patient is asked to pull their left knee toward their chest, as this will posteriorly rotate the innominate bone on that side; this will be the test position. From this position, the therapist looks at the position of the patient's right knee and right ankle. The angular position of the knee to the ankle should be about 90 degrees; a normal length of the right rectus femoris is shown in figure 8.18.

In figure 8.19 the therapist demonstrates the position of the right knee compared with the right ankle. Here, the lower leg is seen to be held in an extended position, which confirms the tightness of the right rectus femoris. You will also notice the position of the hip—it is held in a flexed position. This indicates a tightness of the iliopsoas and was discussed earlier.

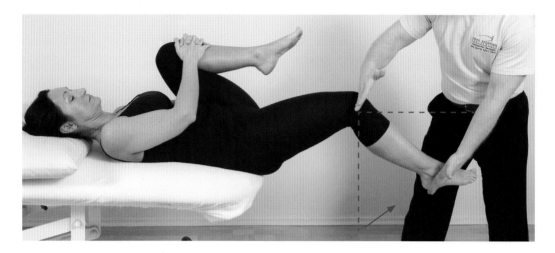

Figure 8.19: The knee is held in extension, indicating a tight rectus femoris.

MET Treatment of the Rectus Femoris

The patient is asked to adopt a prone position, and the therapist passively flexes the patient's right knee until a bind is felt. At the same time, the therapist stabilizes the sacrum with their right hand, which will prevent the pelvis from rotating anteriorly and stressing the lower lumbar spine facet joints.

> **Note:** If you consider the patient to have an increased lumbar lordosis, a pillow can be placed under their stomach. This will help flatten the lordosis and can reduce any potential discomfort.

From the position of bind, the patient is asked to extend their knee against a resistance applied by the therapist (figure 8.20). After a 10-second contraction, and on the relaxation phase, the therapist encourages the knee into further flexion, which will lengthen the rectus femoris, as shown in figure 8.21.

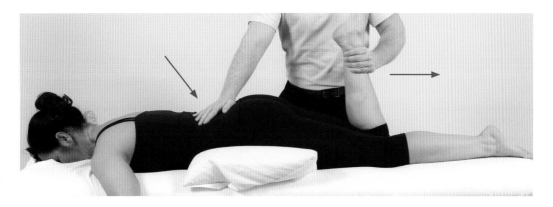

Figure 8.20: The patient extends their knee while the therapist applies resistance.

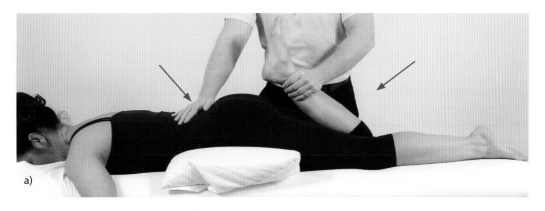

Figure 8.21: The therapist passively flexes the patient's knee to lengthen the rectus femoris while stabilizing the lumbar spine.

Figure 8.22 demonstrates a further lengthening at the origin of the rectus femoris. The initial contraction is exactly the same as depicted in figure 8.20. After the contraction, and on the relaxation phase, the therapist controls the position of the pelvis with their right hand as they slowly flex the knee and extend the hip with their left arm, both at the same time. This will induce a lengthening at the origin and at the insertion of the rectus femoris.

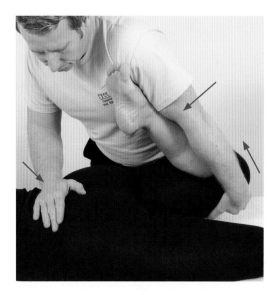

Figure 8.22: The therapist flexes the patient's knee, stabilizes the lumbar spine, and then extends the hip joint.

Alternative MET Treatment of the Rectus Femoris

Some patients may find that the previous MET for the rectus femoris puts a strain on their lower back. An alternative and possibly a more effective MET for the rectus femoris is based on the Modified Thomas Test position.

The patient adopts the position of the Modified Thomas Test as described earlier. The therapist controls the position of the patient's right thigh, and slowly and passively flexes the patient's right knee toward their bottom. A bind will be reached very quickly in this position, so take extra care when performing this technique for the first time.

From the position of bind, the patient is asked to extend their knee against a resistance applied by the therapist (figure 8.23). After the 10-second contraction, and on the relaxation phase, the therapist passively takes the knee into further flexion (figure 8.24). This is a very effective way to lengthen a tight rectus femoris.

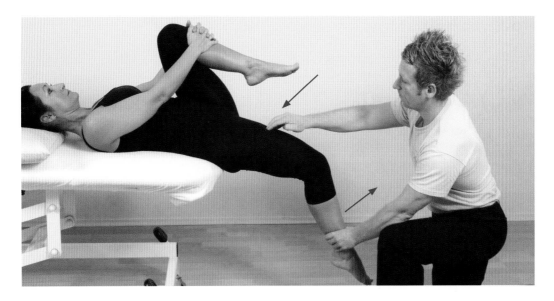

Figure 8.23: The therapist palpates the rectus femoris, and the patient extends their knee.

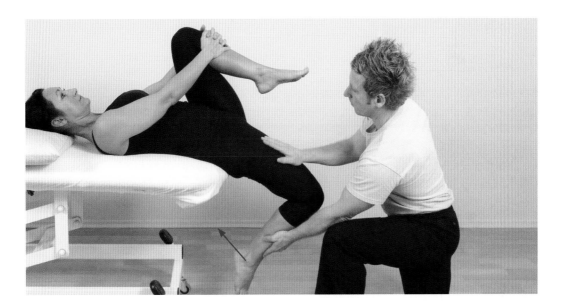

Figure 8.24: The therapist passively flexes the patient's knee to lengthen the rectus femoris.

Tip: Bilateral hypertonicity of the rectus femoris will cause the pelvis to adopt an anterior tilt, resulting in lower back pain due to the fifth lumbar vertebra facet joints being forced into a lordotic position.

Adductors Anatomy

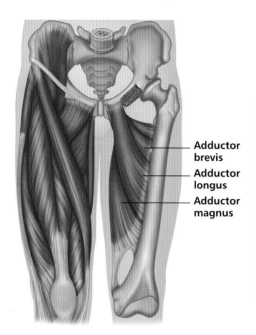

Origin
Anterior part of the pubic bone (ramus). Adductor magnus also has its origin on the ischial tuberosity.

Insertion
Entire length of the medial side of the femur, from the hip to the knee.

Action
Adduct and medially rotate the hip joint.

Nerve
Magnus: Obturator nerve (L2–L4). Sciatic nerve (L4, L5, S1).
Brevis: Obturator nerve (L2–L4).
Longus: Obturator nerve (L2–L4).

— Adductor brevis

— Adductor longus

— Adductor magnus

Figure 8.25: Origin, insertion, action, and nerve innervation of the adductors.

Assessment of the Adductors

Hip Abduction Test
To test the left side, the patient adopts a supine position on the couch. The therapist takes hold of the patient's left leg and passively abducts the hip while palpating the adductors with their right hand (figure 8.26). When they feel a bind, the position is noted; the normal ROM for passive abduction is 45 degrees. If the range is less than this, a tight left adductor group is indicated.

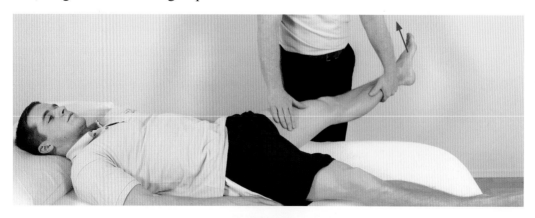

Figure 8.26: The therapist abducts and palpates the adductors for bind.

However, there is an exception to the rule. If the ROM is less than 45 degrees, it could be that the medial hamstrings are restricting the movement of passive abduction. To differentiate between the short adductors and the medial hamstrings, the knee is flexed to 90 degrees (figure 8.27); if the range now increases, this indicates shortness in the medial hamstrings.

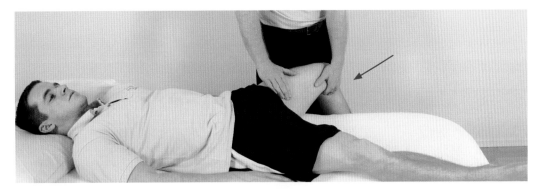

Figure 8.27: The knee is bent to isolate the short adductors.

In summary, to identify if the hamstrings are the restrictive factor, the therapist passively flexes the knee and then continues with the passive abduction, as shown in figure 8.27. If the ROM improves, the hamstrings are the restrictive tissues and not the short adductors.

Note: The term *short adductor* refers to all of the adductor muscles that attach to the femur, the exception being the gracilis. This particular muscle attaches to a point below the knee, on the pes anserinus area of the medial knee, and acts on the knee as well as on the hip.

MET Treatment of the Adductors

One of the most effective ways of lengthening the adductors (short) is to utilize an MET from the position that is demonstrated in figure 8.28. The patient adopts a supine position with their knees bent and heels together; the hips are slowly and passively taken into abduction by the therapist until a bind is felt in the adductors.

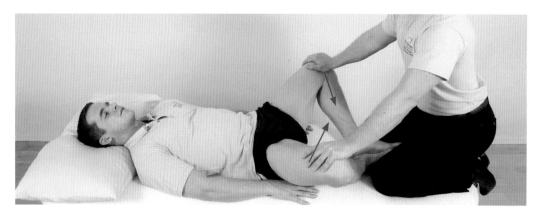

Figure 8.28: The patient adducts their legs against resistance from the therapist.

From the position of bind, the patient is asked to adduct their hips against a resistance applied by the therapist, to contract the short adductors. After a 10-second contraction, and on the relaxation phase, the hips are passively taken into further abduction by the therapist (figure 8.29).

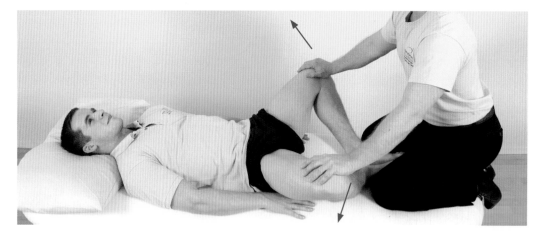

Figure 8.29: The therapist lengthens the adductors.

Tip: Overactivity of the adductors will result in a weakness inhibition of the abductors, in particular the gluteus medius. This can result in a Trendelenburg pattern of gait as explained in chapter 6.

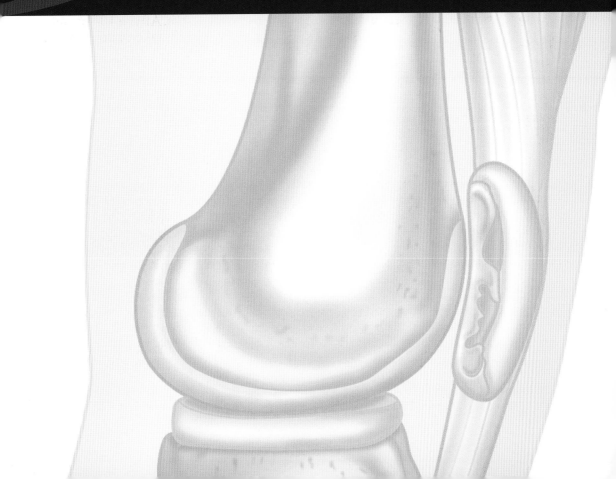

Gmax and Gmed Causing Knee and Ankle Pain

Now think back to the chapter on the gait cycle, as this is the area we need to focus on when trying to decide if the patient's presenting knee or ankle pain is caused by a weakness or misfiring of the glutes.

Knee Anatomy

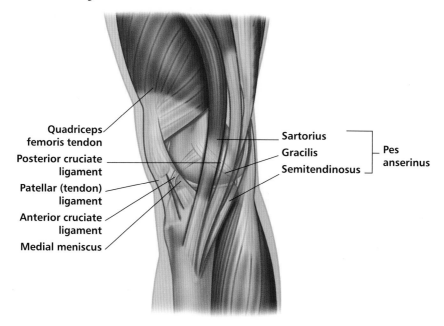

Figure 9.1: The knee joint and associated soft tissue structures.

Common Knee Injuries

There are a multitude of conditions and injuries that affect the knee joint. A common complaint is *patellofemoral pain syndrome (PFPS)*, which causes pain to the anterior aspect of the knee. Some patients may have issues with the internal structures of the knee, such as the meniscus, which helps stabilize the knee. Soccer players and skiers commonly suffer from medial collateral ligament (MCL) sprains. Another common complaint, especially in runners and manifesting in the lateral aspect of the knee, is "runner's knee"; however, we will refer to this condition by its medical name—*iliotibial band friction syndrome*—which relates to the tissue that is responsible for the pain.

Clearly, not all the above-mentioned conditions and injuries result from issues with the glutes. However, since this book is dedicated to maximizing the glutes, the question I ask you is this: *Could* those injuries that relate to the knee joint be a direct, or likelier still an indirect, result of the glutes? If your answer is yes, then the next question I put to you is: *How* can the glutes be responsible for the pain that your patient is presenting with? Have a think about these two questions for a few moments before you read any further.

When I teach physical therapy courses and I focus on the injuries that relate to the knee joint, I generally say to my students or colleagues that when they have patients who present with pain, one has to decide if the pain is purely a "symptom" rather than an actual "cause" of their pain. Out of all the joints in the body, I consider the knee joint in particular to be the weak link in the kinetic chain, but it is commonly not, and I repeat *not*, the underlining cause of the patient's pain.

I often say to my students during lectures that the only person interested or fixated on the area of pain is the patient, for obvious reasons. I do not mean that as a therapist I am not interested in a patient's pain, because clearly it is a vital piece of information. However, beyond its relevance in history-taking, the pain is merely a symptom of underlying dysfunction and is often secondary to the real problem. It is too easy as a therapist to become obsessed with the area of pain rather than trying to determine the underlying cause. It is very tempting to treat only the area of presenting pain, and your patient will expect this. However, if every time you saw your patients you were to focus on and treat only the area of pain, then I can guarantee that the majority of them would not get any better.

You will need to be like a detective and try to work out the location of the dysfunctions and possible weak links that can be responsible for their pain. As Dr. Ida Rolf, who invented the soft tissue technique Rolfing and has taught the physical therapist Tom Myers, states, "Where you think the pain is, the problem is not." I fully understand this statement and I hope that when I lecture, the message is made clear in what I say.

In discussing the following knee syndromes and the potential causes through a weakness of the glutes, I will try my best not to overcomplicate the issue of how and why this weakness can be responsible for pain to the knee joint. I would like my account to be intelligible to all physical therapists, with the aim of helping them achieve a better success rate with their patients.

Gmed and Gmax Causing Iliotibial Band Friction Syndrome

The TFL muscle attaches to the anterior ilium and connects to the ITB, a thick band of connective tissue (fascia) that crosses the hip joint. The ITB extends distally, continuing down the lateral thigh to insert at Gerdy's tubercle on the lateral tibial condyle. It also has an insertion on the lateral patellar retinaculum and on some fibers attaching to the biceps femoris tendon. As you will read later, the ITB has a direct effect on the tracking mechanism of the patellofemoral joint.

What Is Iliotibial Band Friction Syndrome?

Iliotibial band friction syndrome (ITBFS) is a widespread knee injury in athletes, especially those who like to run or cycle. The most common symptom is lateral knee pain resulting from inflammation of the distal portion of the ITB as it crosses the lateral femoral epicondyle. In some athletes, repetitive flexion and extension of the knee results in the distal ITB becoming irritated and inflamed, causing diffuse lateral knee pain. ITBFS can create a lot of frustration in athletes and generally leads to cessation of exercise. Although ITBFS is easily diagnosed clinically, it can be extremely challenging to treat.

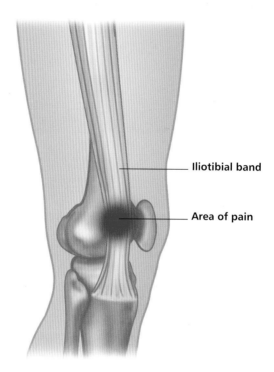

Iliotibial band

Area of pain

Figure 9.2: Iliotibial band friction syndrome (ITBFS).

When a patient presents with ITBFS, the pain is generally localized at the lateral femoral epicondyle, on the lateral side of the knee. Most ITB pain tends to be confined to patients who participate in running and occurs less frequently in those who cycle—hence the name *runner's knee* that is commonly associated with this condition. Patients generally complain of pain at the lateral side of the knee after they have run a certain distance, usually between 2 and 4 km.

It is known that 60–70% of the walking or running cycle is spent on the stance phase, which is restricted to one leg at a time (with 30–40% being spent on the swing phase). If you recall the lateral sling discussion in earlier chapters, we know that the stance phase incorporates the abductors, adductors on the ipsilateral leg, and the QL on the contralateral leg. Let's imagine just for a minute that the adductors are tight and therefore held in a shortened position, and, as a result, the antagonistic group (i.e. the abductors—the Gmed in particular) lengthen through reciprocal inhibition and subsequently weaken. In this case something else needs to take the role of the weak abductors during the stance phase: this is where the TFL enters the equation. Even though it does not want to take the role, the TFL simply has no choice— as I keep mentioning, the body is extremely good at compensating. Once the TFL has adopted its new role, the effect is an increased tension through the ITB, which subsequently causes a potential for friction to occur at the site where it crosses the lateral side of the knee, i.e. the lateral femoral condyle.

Let's look at it from another angle. We know that the function of the muscles inserting into the ITB (TFL) is to abduct the leg. The Gmed, which inserts into the femur, is also an abductor; if this muscle is weak, the ITB will assist in the role of abducting and consequently become overworked. The ITB, however, does not have an insertion that offers a favorable mechanical advantage: in fact, it is at a considerable disadvantage for the purpose of hip and leg abduction activity. Therefore, when the Gmed is weak, the TFL must contract more intensely and over a longer period of time, thus placing extra strain on the ITB.

We know that both the Gmax and the TFL insert into the ITB and are responsible for the stabilization of the lower extremity during the stance phase of the gait cycle. When the Gmax is inhibited, the TFL is left unchecked: this will create a more anterior pull of the ITB over the lateral femoral condyle, which can result in a friction syndrome.

The hip abductors, and in particular the glutes, must support two and a half times the body weight in single-leg stance and significantly more when running. Weakness inhibition of the glutes, which has been related to ankle instability (Beckman and Buchanan 1995), can cause a synergistic dominance of the TFL in frontal plane stabilization of the lower limb; this, as explained above, can lead to a friction syndrome.

A study by Fredericson et al. (2000) corroborates the theory that Gmed weakness is a contributing factor to ITBFS and confirms that retraining for strength gains is an effective treatment. These authors measured hip abductor strength in a group of injured male and female subjects, and found an average deficit of 2% in gluteus medius strength on the injured side compared with the uninjured side. After a six-week retraining program, average hip abductor torque improved by 34.9% in females and 51.4% in males; 22 of the 24 injured athletes were able to return to pain-free running. Most importantly, no injury recurrences were reported at a six-month follow-up.

Gmed Causing Patellofemoral Pain Syndrome

What Is Patellofemoral Pain Syndrome?

Patellofemoral pain syndrome (PFPS) has many names—chondromalacia patellae, anterior knee pain, maltracking syndrome, and retropatellar pain, to give but a few. In simple terms, it is the patellofemoral joint that is causing the patient's pain. The problem lies either in the articular cartilage located within the trochlear groove of the femur, or in the underlying articular cartilage beneath the patella (or possibly in both).

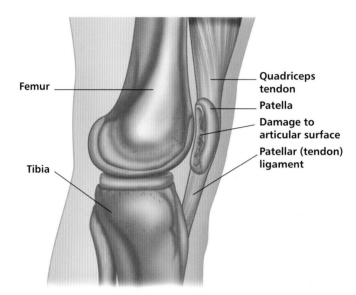

Femur

Tibia

Quadriceps tendon

Patella

Damage to articular surface

Patellar (tendon) ligament

Figure 9.3: Patellofemoral pain syndrome (PFPS).

To understand how this type of pain occurs, an understanding of the structure of the knee joint and the associated patella will be beneficial. The patella is a triangular bone that runs in a groove in the distal aspect of the femur called the *trochlear groove*. The quadriceps tendon inserts superiorly into the patella, and the patella connects inferiorly to the tibial tuberosity by means of a tendon called the *patellar tendon*, known medically as the *ligamentum patellae*. On each side of the fibrous tissue that surrounds the knee joint there are soft tissue attachments called *retinaculae*; the medial side also receives attachments from the insertion of the fibers of the vastus medialis (VM) and the vastus medialis oblique (VMO).

The patella moves within the trochlear groove as the knee flexes and extends. Incorrect tracking of the patella in this groove can cause friction at the sides of the groove, which will eventually lead to pain and inflammation. In most cases of this type of knee pain the patella generally tracks laterally toward the outside of the knee. As a result of the excessive lateral tracking, stress can also be placed on the fibrous tissue on the inside of the knee, which can also be a source of inflammation and pain. Simply put, anything that changes the way the patella moves within the groove can lead to PFPS.

In the discussion on lateral knee pain I mentioned that the ITB has an attachment to the lateral patellar retinaculum. Any increase in tension of the ITB will therefore have an effect on the lateral retinaculum, which will cause a lateral drift of the position of the patella and lead to a maltracking type of syndrome. There is one muscle in the knee joint that is a bit of an anomaly—the VM; what I mean by calling it an anomaly is that this muscle becomes inhibited very quickly when there is pain and swelling present in the joint. Dr. Chris Norris (2011) mentions in his book on sports injuries that it takes only a small amount of fluid—10 mL (~ fl. oz.)—to cause inhibition of the VM, whereas it takes approximately 60 mL to cause inhibition of the rectus femoris. We also know that rehabilitation of the VM is more difficult than one imagines, as I have already said that this muscle does not like to activate in the presence of pain and swelling. Until these two factors are taken out of the equation, the patient will experience ongoing knee pain.

Gmed Causing MCL Pain and Meniscal Pain

There are other factors regarding the Gmed that need to be taken into account when it is a question of medial or lateral knee pain: "medial knee drift," which is a valgus position of the tibiofemoral joint; and, less common, "lateral knee drift," which is a varus position of the tibiofemoral joint. When a patient or athlete consults their physical therapist with knee pain, they might have been told that one of the causes of their knee pain is a weakness found in the Gmax or Gmed. Is it not logical to try to understand the concept of how a weakness of the glutes is responsible for their knee pain? The Gmed posterior fibers assist the Gmax in controlling the alignment of the hip through the knee to the foot during the gait cycle. If for some reason the Gmed posterior fibers are weak, the knee can drift medially when walking or running.

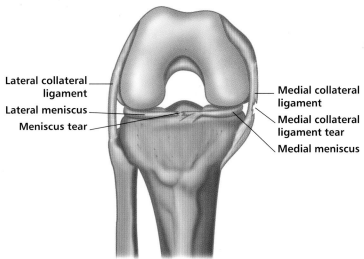

Figure 9.4: The knee joint, showing the meniscus and the MCL.

Which muscle is antagonistic to the Gmed? The answer is the adductors, and if there is an underlying factor that causes the adductors to become tight and shortened, this might in turn be a causative factor for weakness of the Gmed posterior fibers. If the adductors are short, they are generally in a hypertonic state. In this case, when we contact the ground during the gait cycle, the main stabilizing muscle of the lateral sling should be the Gmed, as this also keeps the alignment of the pelvis.

If the adductors receive more neural stimulus from the obturator nerve (as when the adductors have become the main stabilizing muscle instead of the Gmed), this compensation pattern will naturally take the hip into an increased medial rotation, adduction, and hip flexion. As a result, the knee drifts medially (valgus position) because of the increased medial rotation of the femur caused by the hypertonic adductors and the weakened Gmed. As this compensation pattern continues it can be precursory to loading of the MCL and the underlying attachment to the medial meniscus because of the altered biomechanics. Moreover, the lateral meniscus can also be involved owing to a compressive force caused by the increased valgus position of the knee.

Because of the varus position, lateral knee drift is rarely seen in the sports injury clinic. There is limited information in the literature about this condition and many physical therapists may not be aware of it. Lateral knee drift can be observed in a patient performing a single-leg squat if they have a weakness in their Gmed or Gmax. It can also occur when an athlete is running and they have an anterior-tilted pelvis with a forward trunk position. At heel-strike the knee can be forced into a lateral shift so that the Gmed is offloaded and the foot/ankle is forced into a more supinated position. This excessive lateral drift of the knee will place increased strain on the medial meniscus because of the increased compression of the varus position; it can also overload the ITB and the popliteus muscle.

A tight muscle will pull the joint into a dysfunctional position, and a weak muscle will allow it to happen.

Relationship of the Gmed and Gmax to Ankle Sprains

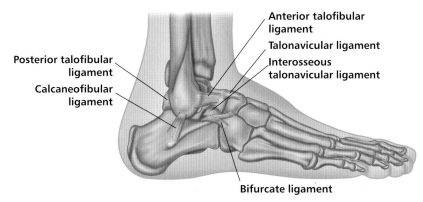

Figure 9.5: The ankle joint, showing the lateral ligaments.

The ankle is the most frequently injured joint, both in athletics and in daily life. Ankle sprains are the most common athletic injury, and 70–85% of these are inversion-type sprains. It has been reported that 10–30% of people with acute inversion-type sprains develop chronic mechanical instabilities as well as functional deficits, and approximately 80% of ankle sprains recur. According to the UK National Health Service (NHS), ankle sprain injuries account for around 1–1.5 million visits to accident and emergency (A&E) departments in the UK each year; it is estimated that every day over 27,000 people in the USA sprain an ankle.

Ongoing recurrent ankle sprains will, over time, lead to chronic ankle instability issues that will then cause kinetic chain dysfunctions. These abnormalities will have a knock-on effect on the homeostasis of the whole body, as the proprioceptive neural senses will now be reduced, and the stability compensatory mechanisms will be altered.

The ankle is a very complex joint comprising the talus, tibia, and fibula bones. The lateral ligaments of the ankle are the most susceptible to injury, and it is estimated that at heel-strike, up to five times the body's weight is loaded onto this joint. The anterior talofibular ligament (ATFL) is generally the most commonly injured, followed by the calcaneofibular ligament (CFL).

Friel et al., in 2006, conducted a study about ipsilateral hip abductor weakness after an inversion ankle sprain; their results showed that hip abduction and plantar flexion were significantly weaker on the involved side. They concluded that unilateral ankle sprains led to weaker hip abduction (Gmed), and suggested exercises to strengthen the hip abductors when developing rehabilitation protocols for ankle inversion sprains.

The influence of a previous ankle sprain in relation to the firing order and timing of the posterior trunk and leg muscles during the hip extension firing test was investigated by Bullock-Saxton et al. in 1994. Those authors found a significant difference in the onset of the Gmax activity (delayed onset) in the group with previous ankle sprains compared with the control group.

In 2010 Leavey et al. reported the results of a study of the comparative effects of balance and strength programs, and a combination of the two, on dynamic postural control. The authors proposed using two types of strategies for maintaining dynamic postural control, specifically a hip strategy and an ankle strategy. For the ankle strategy they suggested utilizing the peroneal muscles to maintain balance, while for the hip strategy the Gmed muscle was recommended for correcting balance and posture. They mention that an individual does not usually strengthen the Gmed muscle when attempting to increase dynamic postural control following a lateral ankle sprain. In most rehabilitation protocols for an inversion sprain, ankle strength training and proprioception training are typically encouraged, as these are used to regain losses in balance that may have occurred. It was also suggested that the weakened Gmed may cause defective dynamic postural control to worsen, leading to the biomechanics of the entire lower extremity becoming altered; this in turn potentially results in faulty movements, making individuals prone to future ankle injuries.

Schmitz et al., in 2002, demonstrated through an EMG study that there was an increase in Gmed activity during sudden ankle inversion in healthy subjects as well as in those with functionally unstable ankles.

Gmax and Gmed Causing Lumbar Spine Pain

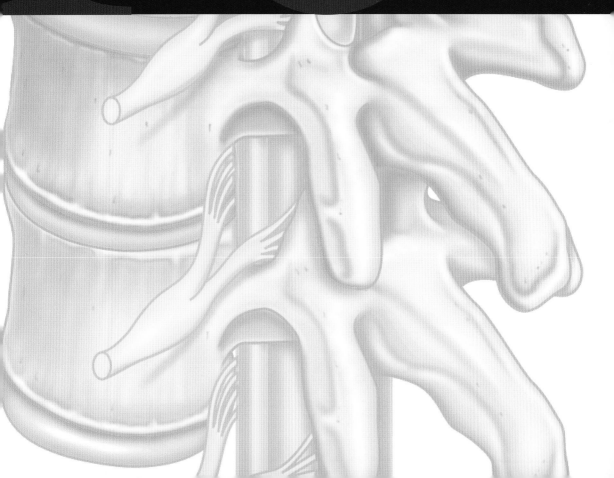

Lumbar Spine Anatomy

Between each of the five lumbar vertebrae there is a structure known as an *intervertebral disc*; in total we have 23 of these structures in the human vertebral column. A disc is made up of three components: a tough outer shell called the *annulus fibrosus*; an inner gel-like substance in the center called the *nucleus pulposus*; and an attachment to the vertebral bodies called the *vertebral end plate*. As we get older, the center of the disc starts to lose water content, a process that will naturally make the disc less elastic and less effective as a cushion or shock absorber.

Nerve roots exit the spinal canal through small passageways between the vertebrae and the discs: such a passageway is known as an *intervertebral foramen*. Pain and other symptoms can develop when a damaged disc pushes into the spinal canal or nerve roots—a condition commonly referred to as a *herniated disc*.

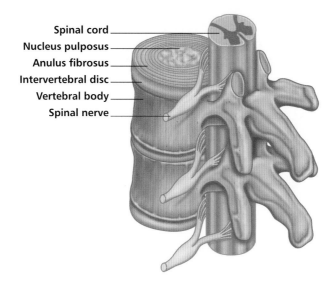

Spinal cord
Nucleus pulposus
Anulus fibrosus
Intervertebral disc
Vertebral body
Spinal nerve

Figure 10.1: Anatomy of the lumbar spine and the intervertebral disc.

Disc Herniation

Herniated discs are often referred to as "bulging discs," "prolapsed discs," or even "slipped discs." These terms are derived from the nature of the action of the gel-like content of the nucleus pulposus being forced out of the center of the disc. Just to clarify, the disc itself does not slip; however, the nucleus pulposus tissue that is located in the center of the disc can be placed under so much pressure that it can cause the annulus fibrosus to herniate or even rupture. The severity of the disc herniation may cause the bulging tissue to press against one or more of the spinal nerves, which can cause local and referred pain, numbness, or weakness in the lower back, leg, or even ankle and foot. Approximately 85–95% of disc herniations will occur either at the lumbar segments L4–L5 or at L5–S1; the nerve compression caused by the contact with the disc contents will possibly result in perceived pain along the L4, L5, or S1 nerve root pathway.

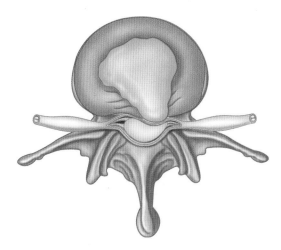

Figure 10.2: Disc herniation.

Degenerative Disc Disease

Degenerative disc disease (DDD) tends to be linked to the ageing process and refers to a syndrome in which a painful disc can cause associated chronic lower back pain, which can radiate to the hip region. The condition generally occurs as a consequence of some form of injury to the lower back and the associated structures, such as the intervertebral discs. A sustained injury can cause an inflammatory process and subsequent weakness of the outer substance of the disc (annulus fibrosus), which will then have a pronounced effect on the inner nucleus pulposus. This reactive mechanism will create excessive movement because the disc can no longer control the motion of the vertebral bodies that are located above and below the disc. This excessive movement, combined with the natural inflammatory response, will produce chemicals that will irritate the local area, which will commonly produce symptoms of chronic lower back pain.

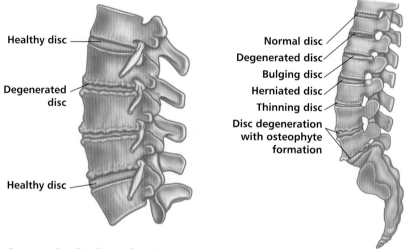

Figure 10.3: Degenerative disc disease (DDD).

DDD has been shown to cause an increase in the number of clusters of chondrocytes (cells that form the cartilaginous matrix and consist mainly of collagen) in the annulus fibrosus (consisting of fibrocartilage). Over a prolonged period of time the inner gelatinous nucleus pulposus can change to fibrocartilage, and it has been shown that the outer annulus can become damaged in areas that allow some of the nucleus material to herniate through, causing the disc to shrink and eventually leading to the formation of bony spurs called *osteophytes*.

Unlike the muscles in the back, the discs of the lumbar spine do not have a natural blood supply and therefore cannot heal themselves; the painful symptoms of DDD can therefore become chronic, eventually leading to further problems, such as discal herniation, facet joint pain, nerve root compression, spondylolysis, and spinal stenosis.

Facet Joint Syndrome/Disease

The facet joints in the vertebral column are located posterior to the vertebral body, and their role is to assist the spine in performing movements such as flexion, extension, side-bending, and rotation. Depending on their location and orientation, the facet joints will allow certain types of motion but restrict others: for example, the lumbar spine is limited in rotation, but flexion and extension are freely permitted. In the thoracic spine, rotation and flexion are freely permitted; extension, however, is limited by the facet joints (but also by the ribs).

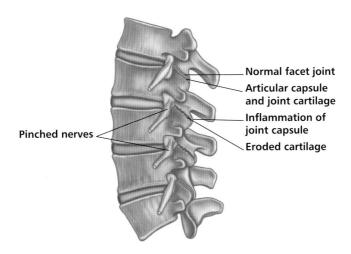

Figure 10.4: Facet joint syndrome.

Each individual vertebra has two facet joints: the *superior articular facet*, which faces upward and works similar to a hinge, and the *inferior articular facet* located below it. The L4 inferior facet joint, for example, articulates with the L5 superior facet joint.

Like all other synovial joints located in the body, each facet joint is surrounded by a capsule of connective tissue and produces synovial fluid to nourish and lubricate the joint. The surfaces of the joint are coated with cartilage, which helps each joint to move (articulate) smoothly. The facet joint is highly innervated with pain receptors, making it susceptible to producing back pain.

Facet joints have a tendency to slide over each other, so they are naturally in constant motion with the spine and, like all types of weight-bearing joint, they can simply wear out and start to degenerate over time. When facet joints become irritated (the cartilage can even tear), this will cause a reaction of the bone of the joint underneath the facet joint to start producing osteophytes, leading to facet joint hypertrophy, which is the precursor of *facet joint disease/syndrome*. This type of syndrome or disease process is very common in many patients presenting with chronic back pain.

Back Pain and Its Relationship to the Glutes

So how and why does weakness of the glutes cause pain to the lumbar spine?

Recall, from the discussion in chapter 3 of the role of the Gmed during the gait cycle, that a weakness of the Gmed can cause either a Trendelenburg or a compensatory Trendelenburg pattern of gait. Think about this, and the possible consequences of this weakness, for a second! As you step onto your left leg, the lateral sling has to come into play: the left Gmed is the main muscle responsible for the control of the height of the right side of the pelvis as you try to stabilize on the left leg. If the Gmed muscle on the left is weak, the pelvis will dip (to the right) as you bear weight. The dipping action will cause the lumbar spine to side bend (to the left) and the facet joints on the left side to compress, as well as the disc and the exiting nerve root, resulting in pain. This side-bending to the left can also cause the iliolumbar ligament on the right side of the spine, as well as other structures such as the joint capsule of the facet joints, to be placed in a stretched position, which can also be a source of pain.

If the left Gmed is weak, the opposite side (right) QL will compensate and work harder as it tries to take on the role of the weak muscle. This increased compensatory pattern will cause over time an adaptive shortening of the right QL that can result in the formation of trigger points and subsequent pain.

Consider the following scenario: a patient presents to the clinic with right-sided QL pain when they walk/run for a certain length of time. The physical therapist palpates the right QL, says it is "tight," and proceeds to release the trigger points that might have developed within the QL. A contract/relax type of technique, such as an MET, might then be used to encourage normality of the length of the QL. The patient and therapist are very happy with the treatment. However, as the patient walks back to their car the QL pain resumes—why? Because a weak left Gmed is forcing the right QL to work a lot harder than it has been designed to do, and the therapist has only treated the presenting symptoms!

Continuing now with the gait cycle, you are now entering the mid-stance phase of gait. This is where the tension of the hamstrings should reduce by the natural anterior rotation of the pelvis and the slackening of the sacrotuberous ligament, and where the Gmax should take the role of extension. However, if the Gmax is weak or misfiring, something else has to take this role; since part of the attachment of the Gmax is on the sacrotuberous ligament, the replacement also needs to be attached to this ligament, as it is part of the force closure mechanism.

A weak or misfiring Gmax might lead to the creation of several compensatory patterns. First of all, let's look at the case when a patient has a weak Gmax, potentially caused by weakness inhibition, commonly known as *reciprocal inhibition* through the antagonistic tightness of the iliopsoas, rectus femoris, and adductors. This soft tissue tightness of the anterior muscles will limit the amount of extension of the hip joint during the gait cycle. As a compensation the innominate bone will be forced to rotate more into an anterior position, and the contralateral innominate will be forced to rotating further into a posterior position. The hamstrings, and in particular the biceps femoris, will be part of the compensation pattern by assisting the increased anterior rotation of the innominate as a result of the weakness of the Gmax. Sahrman in 2002 suggested that if the hamstrings are dominant because of inhibition of the Gmax, an anterior shear of the trochanter can be palpated during the prone leg extension.

This now gets a little complex, as the bit in between the two innominates, i.e. the sacrum, will now have to rotate and side bend a bit more than normal because of the increased innominate rotation. The sacrum will now have to compensate by increasing its torsion (rotation in one direction and side-bending in the opposite direction e.g. rotation left, side-bending right)) in one direction, either a L-on-L sacral torsion (rotation left on the left oblique axis) as seen by fig 10.5a or a R-on-R sacral torsion (rotation right on the right oblique axis) as shown by fig 10.5b. The lumbar spine as shown by the two figures will have to compensate by potentially counterrotating a bit more in the opposite direction to the sacrum.

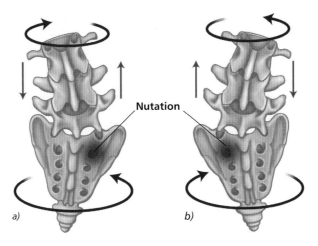

Figure 10.5: Sacral torsion: (a) L-on-L; (b) R-on-R.

There is a natural rotation of the sacral and lumbar spines during the gait cycle; however, because of the increased innominate rotation, the sacrum and lumbar spines have no choice but to compensate as well. In between the lumbar spine and the sacrum (L5 and S1) there lies a disc; imagine now this disc being "torqued" between the two spinal segments. This action will have a negative effect on the disc—it is like squeezing water out of a sponge, and discs do not like that type of increased motion!

Thoracolumbar Fascia and Its Relationship to the Gmax

The thoracolumbar fascia (TLF) is a thick, strong sheet of a ligamentous type of connective tissue, which connects with, and covers, the muscles of the trunk, hips, and shoulders. The normal function of the Gmax will be to exert a pulling action on the fascia, thereby tensing its lower end, as shown in figure 10.6; you can see from the diagram that there is a connection between the Gmax and the contralateral latissimus dorsi muscle by means of the posterior layer of the TLF. Both of these muscles conduct the forces contralaterally (i.e. to the opposite side) during the gait cycle (via the posterior oblique sling), which then causes increased tension through the TLF. This function is very important for rotation of the trunk and for force closure stabilization of the lower lumbar spine and the SIJ.

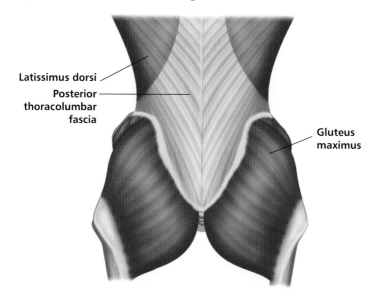

Figure 10.6: The thoracolumbar fascia (TLF) and the connection to the Gmax.

There is also a co-contraction of the deeper muscles of lumbar stability—i.e. the TVA and the multifidus. These muscles co-contract when you move a limb and were discussed in chapter 2. As far as I am aware, there has been nothing published recently about the TVA and multifidus being specifically triggered by engagement of the Gmax. However, I personally think that the TVA muscle definitely responds to Gmax contraction, and I suspect that the multifidus does too, as they all have an association with the sacrotuberous ligament of the pelvis (either directly or indirectly), which assists in force closure of the SIJ.

Hopefully, after reading this chapter you now have an understanding that if the Gmax is weak or misfires, its function of tensing the TLF is reduced, which will cause a natural overactivation of the contralateral latissimus and the ipsilateral multifidus, as well as stimulating other compensatory mechanisms.

Differential Diagnosis of Weakness Inhibition of the Glutes

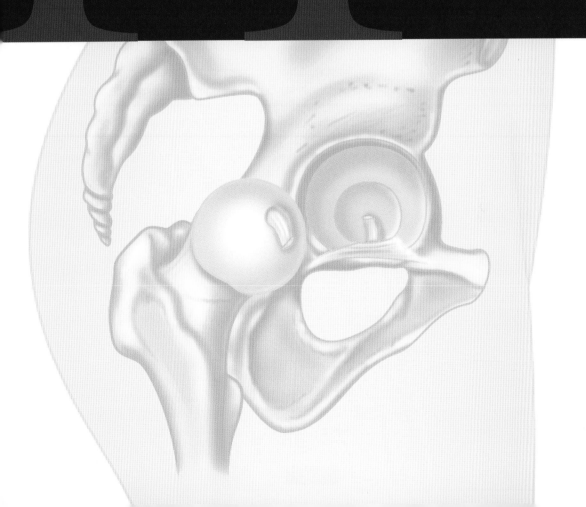

When a patient presents with pain in their body it is the role of the physical therapist to determine whether the pain is the actual cause or a symptom. The therapist also has to decide if the presenting pain is musculoskeletal in origin and not a result of other pathological disease processes.

Having performed a thorough consultation and physical examination, the physical therapist might establish that the Gmax (or possibly the Gmed) tests as weak or exhibits a misfiring sequence. The therapist might then come to the conclusion that this weakness is the main causative factor of the patient's presenting pain.

We have already looked at how the relative shortness of the iliopsoas, rectus femoris, and adductors can be responsible for the apparent weakness inhibition or misfiring of the glutes. These three muscles are antagonistic to the Gmax and Gmed, and because of their anatomical position, any shortness in these muscles can result in a compensatory neurological weakness inhibition of the glutes.

If the therapist determines that the patient's presenting pain is caused by a weakness or misfiring dysfunction pattern, a lengthening program of the iliopsoas, rectus femoris, and adductors should be instigated immediately over a period of no less than two weeks, to see if the patient's symptoms reduce or cease.

However, many times when patients present with pain, and a weakness is suspected to be caused through inhibition of the short antagonistic musculature, even though the patients follow a lengthening program as mentioned earlier, there is no resolution of the symptoms. Why, might one ask? Well, perhaps the weakness is caused by the neurological system, but in a totally different way to that I have suggested throughout this book.

Statistics show that four out of five patients will present with lower back pain at some point in their lives. Some of these patients will have been told that a pain of discogenic origin is responsible for their symptoms on the basis of either a physical examination with specific testing or the results of an MRI (magnetic resonance imaging) scan. Either way, the simple fact is that the intervertebral disc is responsible for their perceived pain. However, one has to be careful here: the issue normally relates to the content of the disc, i.e. the nucleus pulposus, which for some reason has migrated its way through the annulus fibrosus, and is now touching a pain-sensitive structure—for example, the posterior longitudinal ligament—and, more importantly, one of the exiting peripheral nerve roots.

An in-depth study of the neurological system is not within the scope of this book, as I want to keep the discussion simple. I would, however, like to explain a couple of things that might help you to understand this complex but fascinating system.

I already mentioned in chapter 5 that when patients and athletes test positive for weakness or a misfiring of the Gmax or Gmed, for the muscles to contract, the muscle needs a nerve supply to be able to perform this function! Which nerve, I hear you ask? Well, the Gmax is innervated by the inferior gluteal nerve from the 5th lumbar and 1st sacral nerve roots (L5, S1). The level between the 5th lumbar segment and the 1ˢᵗ sacral segment, commonly known as the *L5/S1 disc*, is an important area, as a disc injury here can affect the Gmax. Typically, if there is a disc bulge of some sort at this specific spinal location, the disc content that protrudes can make contact either with the exiting L5 nerve root or, more commonly, with the descending S1 nerve root. When a peripheral nerve root is contacted in this way by a bulging disc, the sensory component of the nerve pathway will be interrupted, which will normally cause a referral pattern of pain to a specific area of the body known as a *dermatome* (see figure 11.1). The disc protrusion can also cause an interruption of the motor component of the nerve as well as the sensory component; this will affect the contractibility of those muscles (including the Gmax) which are served by this nerve, and which are collectively known as a *myotome*.

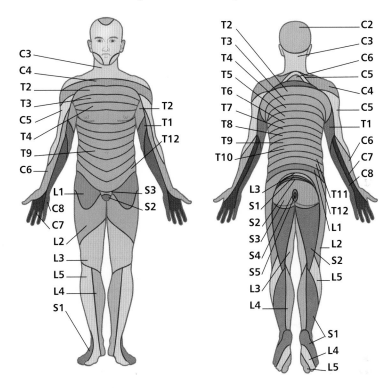

Figure 11.1: Dermatome map of the body.

The S1 myotome is tested through the resisted contraction of the muscles of the Gmax (figure 11.2), gastrocnemius, and peroneals (figure 11.3). However, one must be careful because if the contractile power of only the Gmax is tested, and the same test is not performed on the other two muscles (gastrocnemius and peroneals), one would conclude the Gmax is weak through a possible inhibition of the tight antagonists and not, I repeat *not*, through a neurological dysfunction of the S1 nerve root caused by a potential disc prolapse.

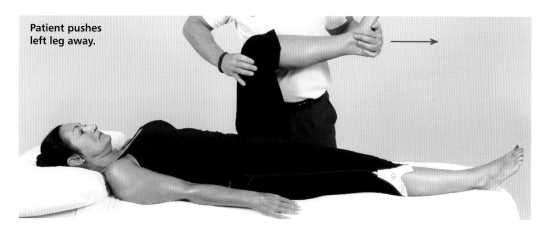

Figure 11.2: The patient contracts the Gmax (S1 myotome).

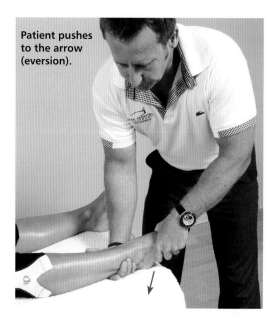

Figure 11.3: The patient contracts the peroneal muscle group (S1 myotome).

However, it is not as simple as that, even though I would like to say it is. What I am trying to say is that when a patient has a disc protrusion that is pressing against any peripheral nerve root, there is usually a referral pattern of pain that tends to originate from the lumbar spine and can manifest itself all the way down the leg and even end up in the foot (sciatica). If you do suspect a nerve root pain coming from the lower level of the intervertebral disc (L5/S1) then you have to be a bit cautious in terms of treatment, as patients commonly have a substantial amount of pain and this might be the cause of the weak Gmax.

Note: If a patient has a disc protrusion touching the motor component of the S1 nerve root, they might be unable to plantar flex their ankle (calf raise movement), because this nerve controls the contraction of the triceps surae (gastrocnemius and soleus).

Another neurological test for differentiating between a weakness of the Gmax from an S1 nerve root compression and an inhibition weakness is the use of a reflex hammer: the Achilles tendon of the gently dorsiflexed foot is tapped to see if there is a normal reflex response from the S1 nerve root (figure 11.4).

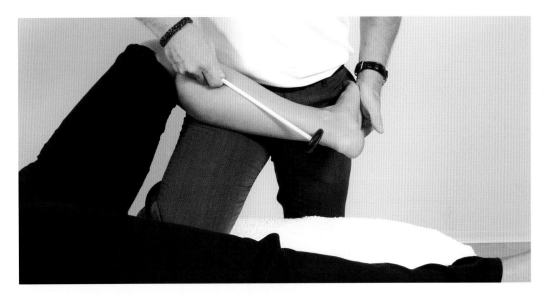

Figure 11.4: Testing the Achilles reflex using a reflex hammer.

As regards the Gmed, the nerve responsible for the contraction of this muscle is the superior gluteal nerve, which originates from the L4/L5 level. One can therefore assume that a confirmed disc protrusion at this location could be the cause of the perceived weakness of the Gmed with an associated Trendelenburg pattern of gait, rather than a short antagonistic muscle of the adductors causing a weakness inhibition.

Note: If a patient has a disc protrusion at the level of L4/5, they might have a weakness in dorsiflexing their ankle (see figure 11.5), since the nerve at this level controls the contraction of the tibialis anterior and extensor digitorum longus.

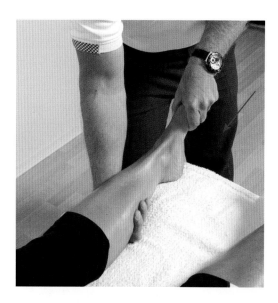

Figure 11.5: The patient contracts the dorsiflexors (L4/5 myotome).

To differentiate between a weakness of the Gmed from an L4 nerve root compression and an inhibition weakness, a neurological test using a reflex hammer can once again be performed: the patellar tendon of the flexed knee is tapped to see if there is a normal reflex response from the L4 nerve root (figure 11.6).

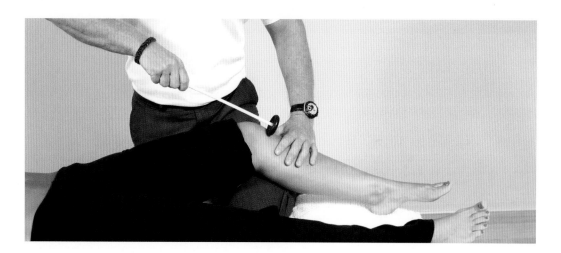

Figure 11.6: Testing the patellar reflex using a reflex hammer.

Hip Capsulitis and the Iliofemoral Ligament

Another possible cause of weakness inhibition of the Gmax is the joint capsule having tightened up: this causes a reflexive spasm in the iliopsoas and hence the weakness inhibition of the Gmax. Today's society is "addicted" to trunk flexion: what I mean by this is that most people tend to sit a lot, drive a lot, and sleep a lot. Think of the common position of the hip joint and trunk during these positions, and the relevance of the anterior structures such as the iliopsoas, hip joint capsule, and iliofemoral ligament (see figure 11.7). All these anterior structures might become compromised in one way or another by adapting to this flexed position.

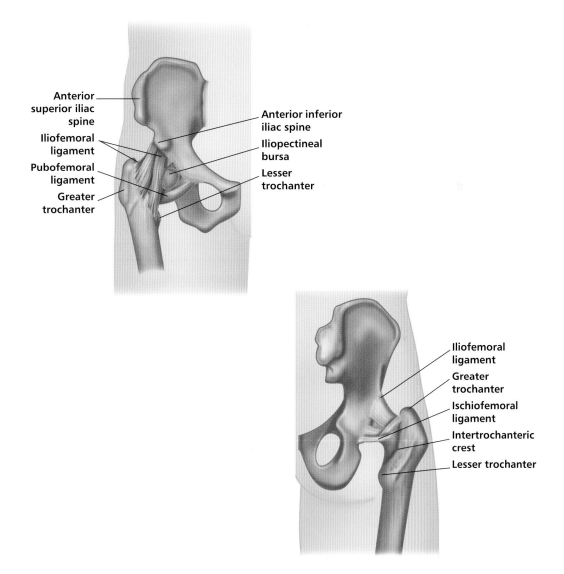

Figure 11.7: Hip joint capsule and the associated structures.

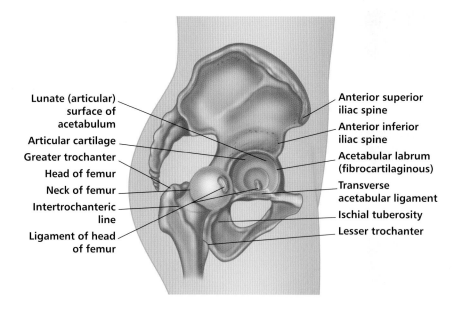

Lunate (articular) surface of acetabulum
Articular cartilage
Greater trochanter
Head of femur
Neck of femur
Intertrochanteric line
Ligament of head of femur

Anterior superior iliac spine
Anterior inferior iliac spine
Acetabular labrum (fibrocartilaginous)
Transverse acetabular ligament
Ischial tuberosity
Lesser trochanter

Figure 11.7: Hip joint capsule and the associated structures.

With a tight iliopsoas a common finding is that the innominate bone is anteriorly rotated on the same side. Imagine, then, a patient with a tight capsule and iliopsoas and an anteriorly rotated innominate on that side. When they walk, the hip has to naturally extend; as they perform this function, the tight structures mentioned will limit the hip extension movement. To try to compensate, the innominate bone will rotate even further into anterior rotation, which will have the effect of switching off the Gmax and switching on the hamstrings, potentially causing microtrauma and tears. At the same time, the opposite side innominate bone will rotate further posteriorly.

As a consequence of all these compensations, the lumbar spine can be forced into an extension position known as a *lordosis*; this increased lordotic position will place extra loading on the facet joints of the lower two lumbar vertebrae (L4/L5), on the facet joints of the 5th lumbar and 1st sacral segments (L5/S1), and on the associated intervertebral discs with the exiting nerve roots.

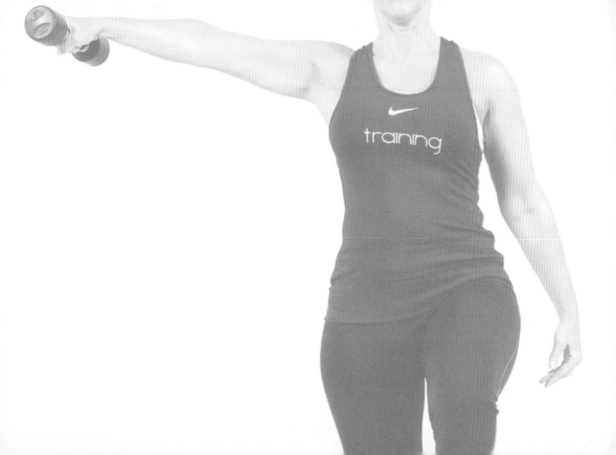

Gmax and Gmed Stabilization Exercises

12

Before discussing the actual stabilization exercises for the Gmax and Gmed, a brief review of the findings of studies that have been carried out in this area will be useful.

Literature Review

Boren et al. (2011) conducted a study involving an EMG analysis of the Gmed and Gmax during rehabilitation exercises performed by 26 healthy subjects. Surface EMG electrodes were placed on the Gmax and Gmed to measure muscle activity during the performance of 18 specific exercises. Maximal voluntary isometric contraction (MVIC) was calculated for each muscle group in order to express each exercise as a percentage of the MVIC and to enable a standardized comparison across subjects to be made. Rank ordering of the exercises was determined using the average per cent MVIC peak activity for each exercise.

The authors concluded that five of the eighteen exercises produced greater than 70% MVIC of the Gmed muscle. In rank order, from the highest EMG value to the lowest, these exercises were:

- Side plank abduction with dominant leg on the bottom (103% MVIC)
- Side plank abduction with dominant leg on top (89% MVIC)
- Single-leg squat (82% MVIC)
- Open clamshell—level 4 (77% MVIC)
- Front plank with hip extension (75% MVIC)

With regard to the Gmax, five exercises recruited that muscle with reported values greater than 70% MVIC. In rank order, from the highest EMG value to the lowest, these exercises were:

- Front plank with hip extension (106% MVIC)
- Gluteal squeeze (81% MVIC)
- Side plank abduction with dominant leg on top (73% MVIC)
- Side plank abduction with dominant leg on the bottom (71% MVIC)
- Single-leg squat (71% MVIC)

Of these latter exercises, all but one (the gluteal squeeze) produced greater than 70% MVIC in both Gmax and Gmed muscles.

A 1999 study by Bauer et al. found that weight-bearing strengthening exercises produce significantly higher Gmed activity than non-weight-bearing exercises. This may be related to the need for increased muscular control owing to the greater external torque forces on the femur and the pelvis.

Earl, in 2005, recommended using the "hip hike" exercise, or standing hip abduction, for the Gmed. In that study the focus was on using open kinetic chain exercises in both the side-lying and standing positions. A blue, or extra-heavy, latex rubber resistance TheraBand was used in the side-lying hip abduction exercise, whereas the standing hip abduction was performed on a multi-hip machine. Two closed kinetic chain exercises, normally performed as part of a lower extremity rehabilitation and/ or strengthening program, were also included, namely single-leg squats and lateral step-downs. Although not found in rehabilitation or strengthening literature for strengthening the Gmed as they are generally regarded as Gmax exercises, these two exercises are often used in a clinical setting.

In 2010 O'Sullivan et al. conducted an EMG study of the three subdivisions of the Gmed in a weight-bearing situation. They analyzed three exercises: static wall squat (WS), pelvic drop (PD), and wall press (WP). A strong relationship was found between the muscle subdivisions of the Gmed and the exercise type. This study demonstrates that the activation of the three subdivisions of the Gmed is significantly different, depending on which one of the exercises is performed. The WP exercise generated the highest EMG amplitudes in all three subdivisions, which suggests that it is an effective isometric strengthening exercise for the Gmed and, in particular, the posterior fibers.

A few other studies with the aim of testing the strength of the Gmed have been carried out on injured subjects with ankle sprains, ITB pain, or PFPS; however, none of these studies offered any suggestions for strengthening the Gmed, even though weakness of that muscle was found to be a contributing factor.

Because of the involvement of the Gmed in dynamic postural control and locomotion during gait, clinicians recommend strengthening this muscle when it is found to be in a weakened state. A study by Ogiwara and Sugiura (2001) suggested the use of progressive resistance exercises (PREs) using a ten-repetition maximum to strengthen the Gmed. PREs have become the most commonly employed method in a clinical and rehabilitation setting for regaining Gmed strength.

The findings of other authors are summarized as follows:

- Distefano et al. (2009): the best Gmed exercises, in order of effectiveness, are side-lying hip abduction, single-leg squat, and single-leg dead lift.

- Distefano et al. (2009): the top exercises, in order of effectiveness, for the Gmax are single-leg squat, single-leg dead lift, and side-lying hip abduction.

- Ayotte et al. (2007): the best exercise for the Gmax is the forward step-up.

- Ayotte et al. (2007): the best exercise for the Gmed is the unilateral wall squat.

- Bolgla and Uhl (2005): the top exercise for the Gmed is the pelvic drop.

Gmed and Side-Lying Abduction

When the Gmed is determined to be weak and misfiring, it is very tempting to try to strengthen it by lifting the leg into abduction while lying on the side as per the test procedure in chapter 6 (figures 6.5 and 6.6). However, if you were to also test for the length and strength of the adductors, TFL, and QL, it is likely that these specific muscles will turn out to be tight and strong. If this is the case then unfortunately the activation of the TFL and QL, rather than the Gmed, would be primarily responsible for the abduction movement (think back to the hip abduction firing pattern test). Remember, too, that the short adductors will probably be "holding" the Gmed weak because of the neurological inhibition process. This means that the two muscles TFL and QL will become stronger and subsequently tighter over time, and the Gmed (which you are trying to strengthen) will actually become weaker as a consequence.

The side-lying abduction is a very common exercise, often performed during "legs, bums, and tums" or "butts and guts" exercise classes. If the goal during this type of class is to strengthen the Gmed (because it is weak and is contributing to, for example, your patient's knee or back pain), unfortunately the Gmed will not, I repeat *not*, get stronger until the lengths of the adductors, TFL, and QL have been normalized.

Gmed and the Use of Orthoses

In 2005 Hertel et al. conducted a study on the effect of foot orthoses on quadriceps and gluteus medius EMG activity during selected exercises. Various orthoses (neutral rear foot post, four-degrees lateral rear foot post, and seven-degrees medial rear foot post), as well no orthosis, were used on three different types of foot position—pes planus (over-pronated), pes cavus (supinated), and pes rectus (neutral). The analysis was carried out for the subjects performing three exercises—lateral step down, single-leg squat, and maximum vertical jump.

The authors found that activation of the Gmed and vastus medialis was greater with the use of all three types of orthosis, regardless of foot position. They concluded that off-the-shelf orthoses could be beneficial in the activation of the Gmed and vastus medialis, regardless of the foot position and type of orthosis used, especially if the single-leg squat and lateral step-down exercises were performed in a slow and controlled manner.

Rehabilitation Methodology

Any rehabilitation program for the Gmax and Gmed should include some if not all of the following exercises. I have split them into *open kinetic chain* exercises and *closed kinetic chain* exercises, beginning with a relatively basic exercise and progressing to ones that are slightly more complex and subsequently more challenging. I consider the exercises to be like a "ladder" system for rehabilitation. If you think of a ladder as a stepping system, then rehabilitation is basically the same concept. We naturally step onto the first rung of the ladder before climbing up the rest: rehabilitation of the glutes can be considered to be a similar process.

> **Definition:** An *open kinetic chain* exercise means that the hand or foot is free to move during the exercise (for example a biceps curl or a hamstring curl). A *closed kinetic chain* exercise means that the hand or foot is fixed and cannot move during the exercise (for example a press-up or a squat).

When the Gmax and Gmed are weak or misfiring they are potentially, in my classification, "clueless" in respect of what functional role they have to play. Glutes that fire normally and are inherently strong will naturally know what job they need to do and when to do it. Strong glutes will know exactly when to switch on to hold the pelvis perfectly level, when to act as shock absorbers, when to abduct and extend the hip, when to fire correctly to keep the trunk, hips, and legs all in correct alignment, and when to contract to propel us forward. These muscles are functionally synergistic to core strength and to a highly functioning posterior and lateral myofascial chain.

I have included the majority of specific exercises that I personally feel will target the muscles of the Gmax and Gmed so that you, the physical therapist, will have a better understanding of how these muscles function to achieve optimal alignment and pelvic stability in your patient/athlete. When the following exercises are performed as I suggest, I truly hope that any pain or dysfunction that your patient might be experiencing somewhere in their body will start to reduce.

You are probably thinking that there are many more exercises which could have been included in the strengthening program. I felt that doing so, however, would have made this book purely a glute exercise book, whereas my goal in writing it was to help the reader understand how to maximize the glutes through other avenues of physical therapy as well as through an exercise program.

Some of the exercises mention the term *dominant leg*. To ascertain the dominant leg, the athlete/patient is asked which foot they consider to be their better kicking foot and that is then judged to be the dominant side. Each exercise is generally performed first with the dominant leg and then repeated with the non-dominant leg.

Reps and Sets

Before embarking on a training program for the glutes, it is important to understand the meaning of the words "rep" and "set." For example, someone may comment that they did three sets of 12 reps on the shoulder press machine. This means that they did 12 consecutive shoulder presses, had a break (rest), and then repeated the process a further two times.

> **Definition:** A *rep* (or repetition) is one complete motion of an exercise. A *set* is a group of consecutive repetitions.

There is no simple answer to the question of how many reps and sets should be performed, as the number of reps required depends on many factors, including where the patient/athlete is in their current training and what their individual goals are. Remember, the purpose of this book is to improve the optimum functionality of the glutes so that your patient/athlete can perform the activities needed for everyday life, as well as participate in any sports-related activities. I suggest we aim for between 10 and 12 repetitions and between one and two sets of each exercise, at least to start with.

Please also remember that, as with any training program, the work-outs will need to be progressive. For example, let's say the patient starts with four exercises that I have chosen from the open-chain section and they perform two sets of 10 reps for each exercise; when the patient gets to the stage where they find these exercises to be relatively easy, it is then time to progress. This might happen after one week or it might take longer, perhaps three or four weeks. The exercise can be made more difficult by simply changing the number of reps, reducing the rest period between sets, or adding in another exercise. To progress in the program, you could, for example, ask the patient to either increase the number of reps, i.e. perform two sets of 12 reps (instead of 10 reps), or rest for only 30 seconds (instead of 45 seconds) between the sets. I highly recommend that everything is written down, as it is very easy to forget what was done on the previous training session—trust me on this! I can guarantee that within a few weeks the patient/athlete will easily be doing three sets of 12 reps for six or seven different types of gluteal exercise.

The following exercises do not specify the number of reps and sets next to the exercise diagram, as I want to demonstrate how to perform the individual exercises correctly. Refer to the appendix for a "Gmax and Gmed Stabilization Exercise Sheet:" the blank boxes allow you to record the number of reps and sets for your patient's rehabilitation program.

> **Important note:** Please be aware that some of the following exercises, notably the Side/Front Plank, can cause an increase in pressure in the patient's body, especially if they have a tendency to hold their breath. If there is any history of spinal disc pathology, or even blood pressure issues, extra care must be taken when attempting any of the following exercises. It is recommended that the patient seek the advice of a medically trained professional before starting any strengthening program, and not just performing gluteal-specific exercises.

Open Kinetic Chain Exercises

Open kinetic chain (OKC) exercises are rehabilitation techniques employed where the hand or foot is not fixed and is free to move during the exercise. Most physical therapists and trainers employ OKC exercises, especially in a sports complex or a clinical setting, to strengthen the glutes, and in particular the Gmed. These types of movement tend to isolate a single muscle group and a single joint; because of this factor, OKC exercises have also been termed *non-functional* exercises.

Generally, the Gmed is strengthened using a side-lying straight leg raise as the hip is moved into abduction. This is usually performed against an elastic resistance or an ankle cuff weight, and is very common in some exercise classes. Pilates trainers advise another type of open-chain exercise for the Gmed—the "open clam," for which the client/patient again adopts a side-lying position with their legs stacked and a neutral position of the lumbar spine, but this time with the hips flexed to 45 degrees and the knees flexed to 90 degrees.

The open clam is still regarded as the king of all exercises for strengthening the Gmed, especially in a rehabilitation and clinical setting. I think this exercise is more effective, however, in the early phase of rehabilitation, as the exercise is open chain, which I consider to be of limited benefit for functional stability of the weight-bearing phase of the gait cycle.

Open Clam Exercise

Level 1
The patient lies on their non-dominant side, with their hips flexed to approximately 45 degrees, knees flexed to 90 degrees, and feet together, as shown in figure 12.1(a). While keeping their heels together and maintaining activation of their core muscles, the patient is instructed to externally rotate their top leg to bring the knees apart, as shown in figure 12.1(b). This movement will induce hip abduction with an external rotation. The patient is advised to stop the movement when they feel their pelvis position change and it starts to rotate; this is normally around 45 degrees. The patient is then asked to hold this position for 2 seconds (count of two) before returning to the starting position. Once the patient is capable of performing level 1 with ease, they can proceed to the next level.

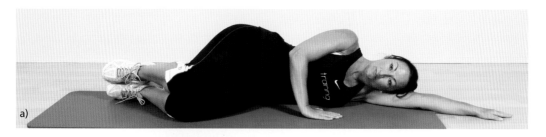

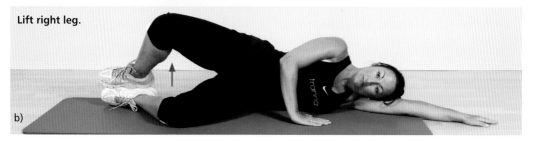

Figure 12.1: Open Clam: (a) Level 1—start position; (b) Level 1—finish position.

Level 2

Maintaining the same position as in level 1 (figure 12.1(a)), the patient is instructed to keep their knees together while internally rotating the top hip to lift the top foot away from the bottom foot until they reach a position of bind (figure 12.1(c)), before returning to the start position.

> **Note:** A restriction or a feeling of bind experienced by the patient when performing the motion of internal rotation can be due to a pathological change in the hip joint, for example capsulitis or even a degenerative process of OA.

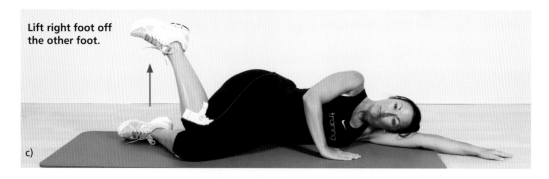

Figure 12.1: (c) Level 2—position of bind.

Level 3

The start position is the same as in level 2, but with the top leg raised parallel to the floor (see figure 12.1(d)). Maintaining the height of the knee, the patient internally rotates at the hip by lifting their foot toward the ceiling (figure 12.1(e)) until a bind is felt, before returning to the start position. The patient is then asked to externally rotate the hip until a bind is felt (figure 12.1(f)), before lowering the leg back to the floor to rest.

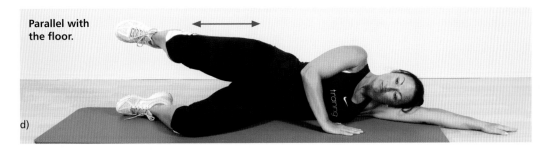

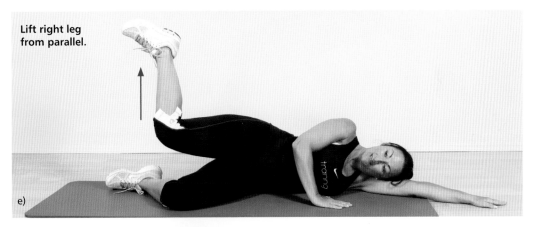

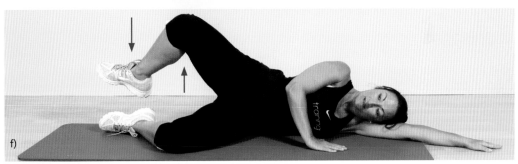

Figure 12.1: (d) Level 3—start position; (e) Level 3—internally rotated position; (f) Level 3—externally rotated position.

Level 4

The patient positions themselves as in level 3, but with the hip joint at full extension (see figure 12.1(g)). As in level 3, the patient maintains the height of the knee and externally rotates at the hip by turning their foot toward the ceiling (figure 12.1(h)) until a bind is felt, before returning to the start position.

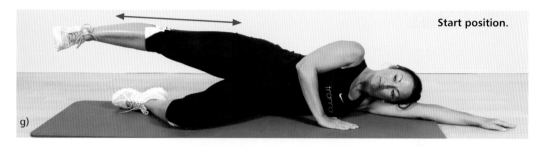

Start position.

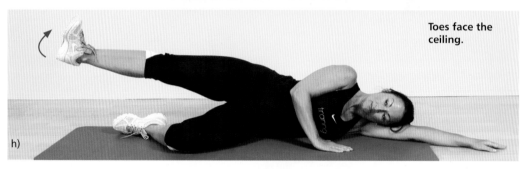

Toes face the ceiling.

12.1: (g) Level 4—hip fully extended, start position; (h) Level 4—hip fully extended, externally rotated position.

Side-Lying Hip Abduction

Level 1

The patient adopts a side-lying position on the non-dominant side. Maintaining a neutral position of the hip and lumbar spine, the patient is then instructed to flex the hip and knee of the support side, as shown in figure 12.2(a). Once the patient has adopted this position they are then asked to abduct the dominant leg to approximately 30 degrees while maintaining neutral spine with the toes pointing forward, as shown in figure 12.2(b), before returning to the start position.

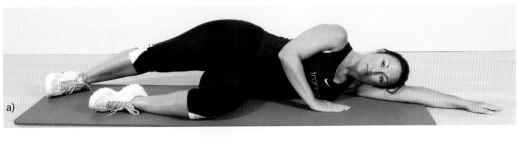

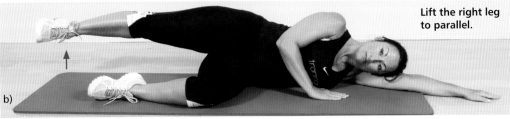

Lift the right leg to parallel.

Figure 12.2: Side-Lying Hip Abduction: (a) Level 1—start position; (b) Level 1—finish position.

Level 2

The patient adopts a side-lying position as in level 1. The only difference this time is that the patient is instructed to bring their dominant hip into slight extension and external rotation, so that their toes are pointing slightly toward the ceiling to activate the posterior fibers of the Gmed, as shown in figure 12.2(c). Once they have adopted this position they are asked to abduct their leg to approximately 30 degrees while maintaining this position of the hip and toes, as shown in figure 12.2(d), before returning to the start position.

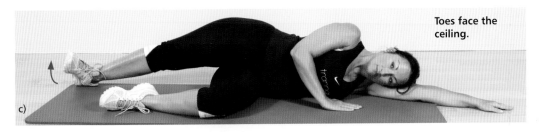

Toes face the ceiling.

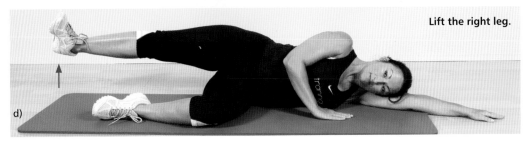

Lift the right leg.

Figure 12.2: (c) Level 2—start position; (d) Level 2—finish position.

Side Plank

Level 1

The patient adopts a side-lying position with the dominant leg up. Keeping their shoulders, hips, knees, and ankles in line bilaterally, the patient is instructed to rise into a side plank position, with their hips lifted off the floor to achieve neutral alignment of the trunk, hips, and knees (figure 12.3(a)). Allowing their upper torso to be used as support, the patient is asked to maintain the plank position while balancing on their elbows and feet.

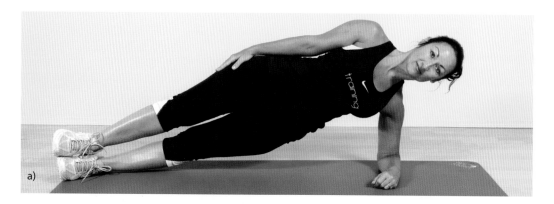

Figure 12.3: Side Plank: (a) Level 1—neutral alignment in raised position.

Level 2

The patient assumes a side plank position as in level 1, with the dominant leg up (figure 12.3(a)). While balancing on their elbows and feet, the patient raises their top leg into abduction for 2 seconds (one repetition), as shown in figure 12.3(b). The patient is instructed to maintain the plank position throughout all repetitions.

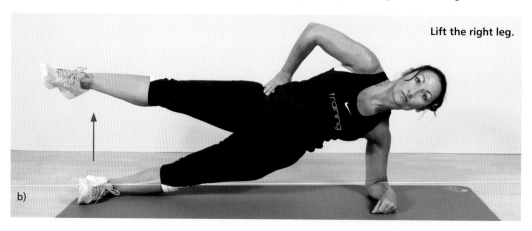

Figure 12.3: (b) Level 2—with abduction.

Hip Extension on All Fours

Level 1

The patient starts in a position on all fours (figure 12.4(a)). They are instructed to extend their dominant leg at the hip, while keeping their knee flexed 90 degrees as the foot is lifted toward the ceiling, as shown in figure 12.4 (b). The foot is lifted to achieve neutral hip extension, before returning to the start position.

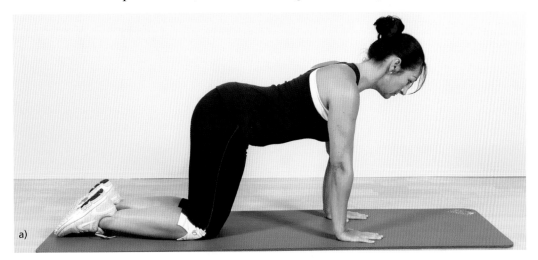

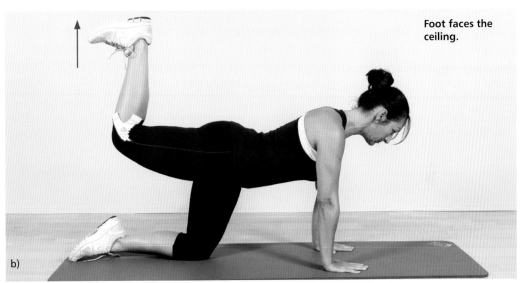

Foot faces the ceiling.

Figure 12.4: Hip Extension on All Fours: (a) Level 1—start position;
(b) Level 1—foot is lifted toward the ceiling.

Level 2

The patient adopts the position on all fours as in level 1 (figure 12.4(a)). They are instructed to extend the dominant leg at the hip, but this time keep their knee in extension as they lift their heel toward the ceiling (figure 12.4(c)), before returning their leg to the start position. The fully extended position of the leg in this exercise increases the leverage to the glutes.

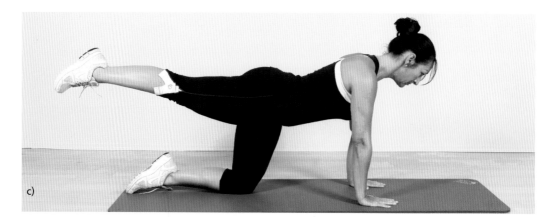

c)

Figure 12.4: (c) Level 2—hip and knee in extension.

Front Plank

Level 1

The patient adopts a prone position, resting on their elbows in a plank position with their trunk, hips, and knees in neutral alignment, as shown in figure 12.5(a). The patient is asked to maintain this position while activating their inner core and gluteal muscles for a specified period of time: for example, they could begin with 10 seconds and work up to 15 seconds and so on until they achieve the desired time.

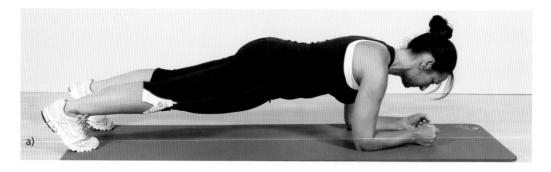

a)

Figure 12.5: Front Plank: (a) Level 1—maintaining the plank position.

Level 2
Starting from the plank position in level 1 (figure 12.5(a)), the patient is asked to lift their dominant leg off of the floor for a count of two seconds (figure 12.5(b)), before returning to the start position.

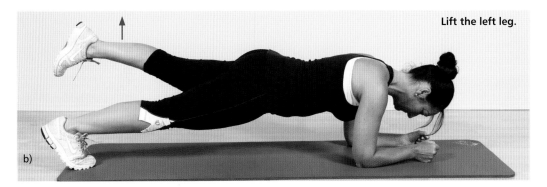

Figure 12.5: (b) Level 2—with hip extension.

Closed Kinetic Chain Exercises

Closed kinetic chain (CKC) exercises are rehabilitation techniques employed where the hand or foot is fixed and cannot move, which means that either the hand or the foot is in contact with an immobile surface, such as the floor. CKC exercises are thought to be more functional in the rehabilitation process, and some authors state that these exercises are utilized more frequently in the rehabilitation setting as they are considered safer. CKC exercises are generally compound movements that incorporate multi-joint planes of motion: for example, a squat exercise will incorporate motion from the lumbar spine, pelvis, hip, knee, ankle, and foot. An exercise that includes all these specific areas of the body is considered to be a functional exercise, since they are involved in normal day-to-day activities as well as playing a part in a sporting environment. CKC exercises, as explained, will involve more than one joint and simultaneously incorporate more than one muscle group, rather than focusing on only one joint motion as in the case of OKC exercises.

CKC exercises, when incorporated into the rehabilitation program, can impose a "compressive" type of force on the joints, whereas OKC exercises can potentially place a "shearing" type of force on the joint. Nonetheless, OKC and CKC exercises naturally co-exist in any form of strengthening or rehabilitation program.

Dissociation Pattern in Lying

The following two initiation exercises are basically open chain; however, I like to add these specific exercises early on in a program, as I want the patient/athlete to be able to feel the exact area that I wish them to be working, before they progress. The patient needs to be aware of which muscle(s) is being worked, as well as actually feel the muscle working. I find it helpful to teach some basic anatomical knowledge to the people I am looking after, so that they understand the strengthening process.

Gluteal Squeeze (Lying)

The patient lies prone, with their feet shoulder-width apart and their hands lightly placed on their glutes. They are then asked to maximally contract their right glute and hold for 2 seconds (figure 12.6(a)), before relaxing and repeating on the left side. Once the patient is able to dissociate the left glute from the right one at least five times in succession, they are asked to maximally contract both glutes. The contraction is held for 2 seconds (figure 12.6(b)) and then a rest taken for 2 seconds, before repeating for the desired number of reps.

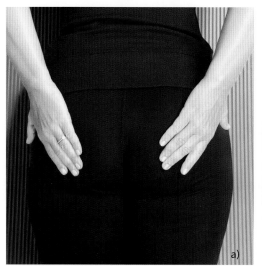 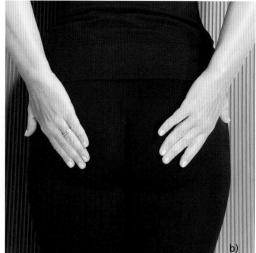

Figure 12.6: Gluteal Squeeze (Lying): (a) Right glute only; (b) Bilateral.

Squeeze and Lift

The patient lies prone with their feet shoulder-width apart and their hands either lightly placed on the glutes or resting by the side of the head. They are asked to maximally contract their right glute (figure 12.6(a)). Once they have the contraction they are instructed to lift the right leg 2" off the couch, and hold the position for 2 seconds, as shown in figure 12.6(c). The patient then rests for 2 seconds, before repeating on the left leg.

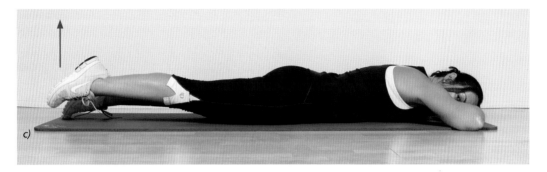

Figure 12.6: (c) Right glute with lift.

Progression 1: Pelvic Tilt

The patient assumes a supine position, with their hips flexed to 45 degrees, their knees bent to 90 degrees, and their spine maintained in what is termed a *neutral position*, as shown in figure 12.7(a). They are then instructed to tilt their pelvis in anterior and posterior directions, which will cause the lumbar spine to flex and extend. Perhaps a more descriptive instruction is to tell your patient to "arch the lower back" and then to "flatten the back." The glutes will be responsible for the flattening component (posterior pelvic tilt) of the lumbar spine, so ask the patient to maximally contract their glutes when they flatten their back, as shown in figure 12.7(b). This position is held for 2 seconds and then repeated as necessary.

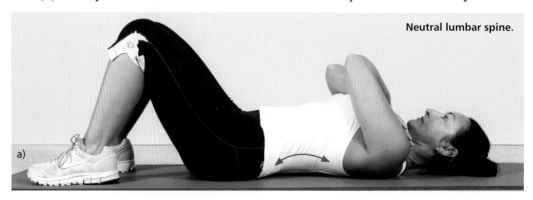

Neutral lumbar spine.

a)

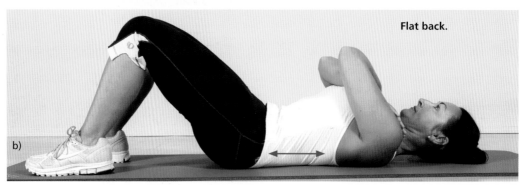

Flat back.

b)

Figure 12.7: Pelvic Tilt: (a) Neutral position of the lumbar spine; (b) Flattening the back.

Progression 2: Pelvic Lift

The patient adopts the same position as described for the pelvic tilt, maintaining a neutral position of the lumbar spine. For this progression, the hands are placed next to the glutes (the patient can also be instructed to palpate the glutes lightly if preferred, so that they are aware of the activation) (figure 12.8(a)). The patient is asked to lift their hips off the floor by using *only* their glutes, and is told not to activate their hamstrings. Provided the patient has engaged just the glutes, the hips can be lifted a few inches off the floor and this position held for 2 seconds, as shown in figure 12.8(b), before lowering down to the start position.

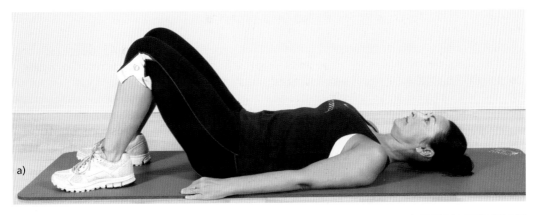

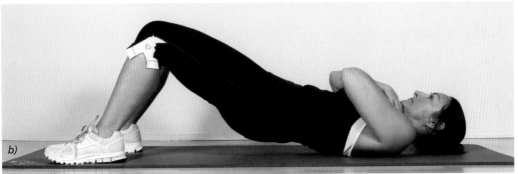

Figure 12.8: Pelvic Lift: (a) Start position; (b) Raised position.

Progression 3: Bridging on a Stable Surface

The patient begins in the same position as for progression 1 (figure 12.7(a)). They are then instructed to lift their pelvis up into a "bridge position" on both legs. Keeping their feet on the floor, the patient raises their hips to achieve neutral alignment of the trunk and hips, while maintaining 90-degree knee flexion, for 2 seconds, as shown in figure 12.9, before lowering the body down to the floor to the start position.

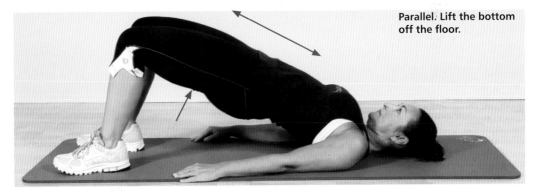

Parallel. Lift the bottom off the floor.

Figure 12.9: Bridging on a Stable Surface.

Progression 4: Single-Leg Bridging on a Stable Surface

The patient begins in the same position as for progression 1 (figure 12.7(a)). They are then instructed to lift their pelvis up into the bridge position on both legs by keeping their feet on the floor and raising their hips to achieve neutral alignment of the trunk and hips, while maintaining 90-degree knee flexion (figure 12.9). From this position, the patient is asked to extend the knee of the non-dominant leg to full knee extension while keeping both femurs parallel, as shown in figure 12.10. The patient holds this position for 2 seconds and returns the non-dominant leg to the bridge position. The full knee extension movement is repeated on the dominant leg side, before lowering the body down to the floor. The patient should be able to feel muscle activation in the glutes and not in the hamstrings.

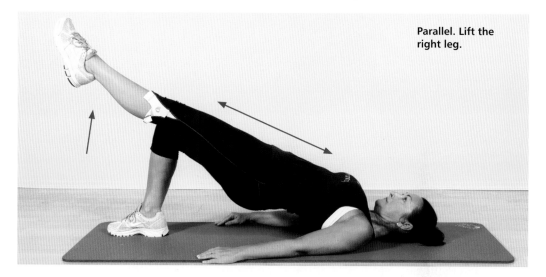

Parallel. Lift the right leg.

Figure 12.10: Single-Leg Bridging on a Stable Surface.

Balance Stabilization

Balance is generally considered to be a static component of fitness; however, functional balance is a dynamic stabilization process involving multiple neurological components. Gmax and Gmed strength-based training should be incorporated into any form of functional training program.

Level 1: Dissociation Pattern in Standing

Gluteal Squeeze (Standing)

This exercise is similar to the Gluteal Squeeze (Lying) exercise, except that the patient now stands with the feet shoulder-width apart. With their hands lightly placed on their glutes, the patient is then asked to maximally contract their right glute and hold for 2 seconds (figure 12.11(a)), before relaxing and repeating on the left side. Once the patient is able to dissociate the left glute from the right one at least five times in succession, they are asked to maximally contract both glutes. The contraction is held for 2 seconds (figure 12.11(b)) and then a rest taken for 2 seconds, before repeating for the desired number of reps.

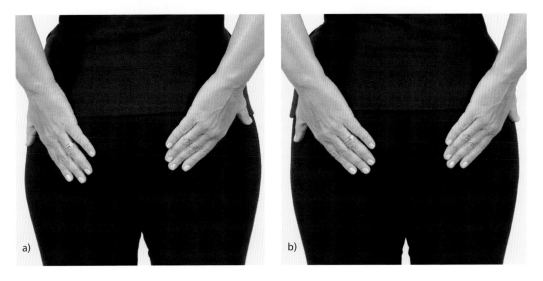

Figure 12.11: Gluteal Squeeze (Standing): (a) Right glute only; (b) Bilateral.

Level 2: Balance

Alternate Standing on One Leg

The patient stands with their legs about shoulder-width apart, as shown in figure 12.12(a). They are asked to engage the weight-bearing dominant-side Gmed and instructed to lift the non-dominant leg just off the floor, as shown in figure 12.12(b). This position is held for 5 seconds, before returning the leg to the start position. The time is increased from 5 seconds to 10 seconds and so on, until the patient can manage 30 seconds with ease using either leg.

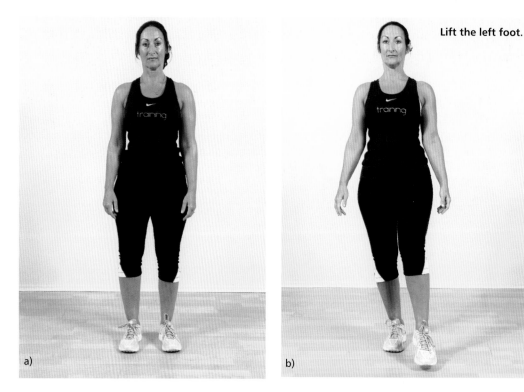

Figure 12.12: Alternate Standing on One Leg: (a) Start position; (b) Leg raised off the floor.

As the patient performs the Alternate Standing on One Leg exercise, the therapist should look out for the following principal faults:

1. Excessive lateral shift to the weight-bearing leg.

2. Dipping of the pelvis to the contralateral side (which might indicate a Trendelenburg pattern of gait).

3. Instability of the weight-bearing leg (a proprioception issue with the ankle complex, or a weakness of the glutes).

4. Medial or lateral knee drift.

If any of these four dysfunctional patterns are observed, a potential weakness within the Gmed could be indicated.

Progression 1: Sagittal Plane One-Leg Swing

The patient stands on their dominant leg and maintains a balanced position (figure 12.12(b)). They are instructed to slowly bring their non-dominant leg forward and backward, as shown in figures 12.13(a) and (b). This flexion and extension movement of the hip joint will challenge the Gmed in the sagittal plane of motion. The exercise is initially performed for 3 reps, before swapping legs to work the non-dominant side. Once this is comfortable, the patient moves on to 5 reps, and gradually works up to 10.

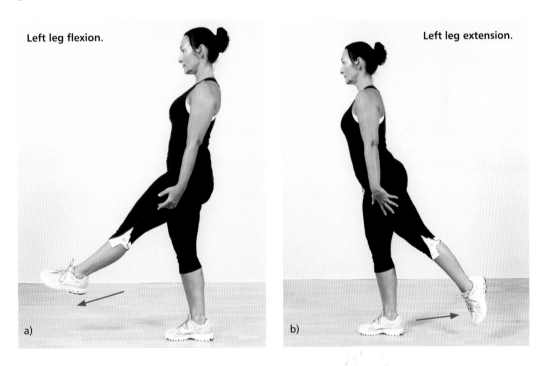

Left leg flexion.

Left leg extension.

a)

b)

Figure 12.13: Sagittal Plane One-Leg Swing: (a) Flexion; (b) Extension.

Progression 2: Frontal Plane One-Leg Swing

The patient stands on their dominant leg and maintains a balanced position (figure 12.12(b)). They are instructed to slowly swing their non-dominant leg to the side, away from the body and back toward the body, as shown in figures 12.14(a) and (b). This abduction and adduction movement of the hip joint will challenge the Gmed in the frontal plane of motion. The exercise is performed for 3 reps, before swapping legs to work the non-dominant side.

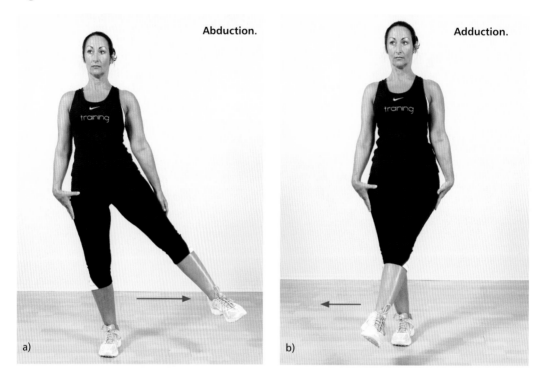

Figure 12.14: Frontal Plane One-Leg Swing: (a) Abduction; (b) Adduction.

Progression 3: Transverse Plane One-Leg Rotation

The patient stands on their dominant leg and maintains a balanced position (figure 12.12(b)). They are asked to slowly lift their non-dominant hip and knee to 90 degrees, as shown in figure 12.5(a). From this position, the patient is instructed to rotate their non-dominant hip to the right and then back to the left, as shown in figures 12.15(b) and (c). This rotational movement of the hip will challenge the Gmed in the transverse plane of motion. The exercise is performed for 3 reps, before swapping legs to work the non-dominant side.

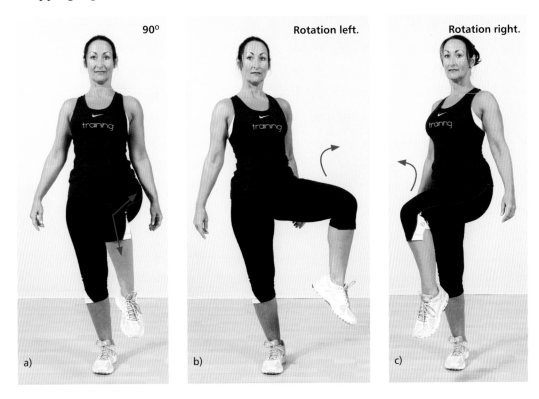

Figure 12.15: Transverse Plane One-Leg Rotation: (a) Start position; (b) Rotation left; (c) Rotation right.

Progression 4: Hip Circles on a Stable Surface

The patient stands on their dominant leg and maintains a balanced position (figure 12.12(b)). They are asked to place the toes of the non-dominant leg laterally over an imaginary point on the floor (starting position). Slightly bending the knee of the dominant leg to maintain balance control, the patient is then asked to trace the toes of the non-dominant leg around an imaginary circle for one revolution, as shown in figure 12.16, until the foot is back at the starting position.

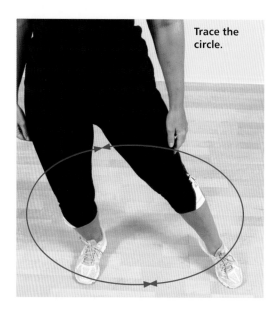

Figure 12.16: Hip Circles on a Stable Surface.

Level 3: Balance with Coordination

To progressively rehabilitate the glutes we need to add exercises that are more challenging, since the patient is consciously controlling the activation of the Gmed when they are asked to stand on one leg. If we add in movements that are more complex, the patient will control the motion of, for example, the arms by a conscious action, whereas the glutes will now stabilize the pelvic position through a subconscious action.

Single-Leg Stance with Ipsilateral Arm in Two Planes
The patient stands on the dominant leg and lifts the other leg a few inches off the floor, as shown in figure 12.17(a). Once this position is maintained, the patient is instructed to lift their ipsilateral arm into flexion (sagittal plane movement) and abduction (frontal plane movement) for 10 reps, as shown in figures 12.17(b) and (c). The ipsilateral arm lift means that the patient lifts the arm on the same side as the weight-bearing leg (dominant side).

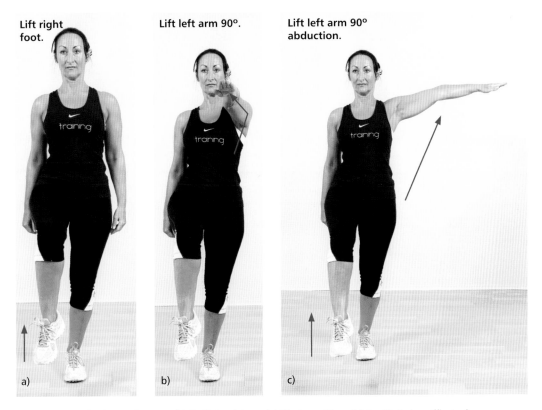

Figure 12.17: Single-Leg Stance with Ipsilateral Arm: (a) Start position; (b) Sagittal plane (flexion); (c) Frontal plane (abduction).

Progression 1: Single-Leg Stance with Contralateral Arm in Two Planes

The patient stands on the dominant leg and lifts the other leg a few inches off the floor (figure 12.17(a)). Once this position is maintained, the patient is instructed to lift their contralateral arm into flexion (sagittal plane movement) and abduction (frontal plane movement) for 10 reps, as shown in figures 12.18(a) and (b). The contralateral arm lift means that the patient lifts the arm on the opposite side to the weight-bearing leg (dominant side), which makes the exercise more challenging for the Gmed.

Lift left arm and leg.

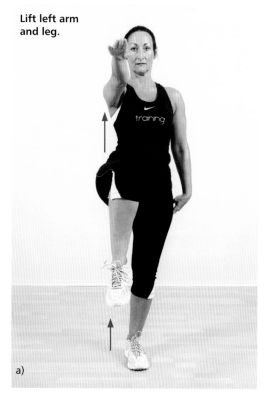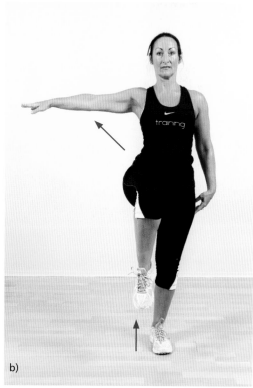

a)

b)

Figure 12.18: Single-Leg Stance with Contralateral Arm: (a) Sagittal plane (flexion); (b) Frontal plane (abduction).

Progression 2: Single-Leg Stance with Ipsilateral/Contralateral Arm in Two Planes—with Weight

The patient stands on the dominant leg and lifts the other leg a few inches off the floor while holding a weight, as shown figure 12.19(a). Once this position is maintained, the patient is instructed to lift their ipsilateral arm into abduction and flexion for 10 reps, as shown in figures 12.19(b) and (c). This is then repeated with the contralateral arm, as shown in figures 12.19(d) and (e). Lifting the contralateral arm (the arm opposite to the weight-bearing leg) makes the exercise more challenging for the Gmed.

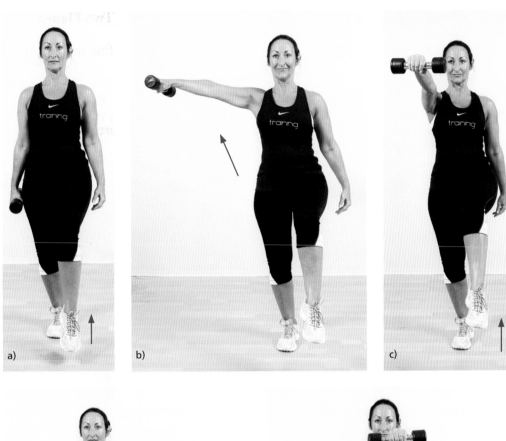

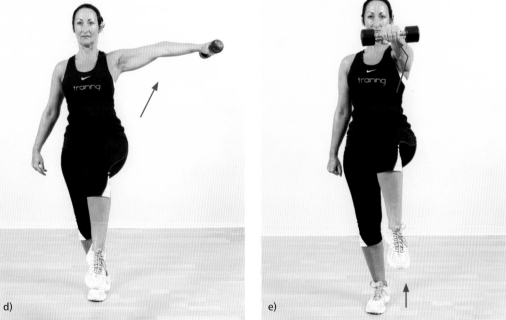

Figure 12.19: Single-Leg Stance with Weight: (a) Start position; (b) Ipsilateral arm—frontal plane (abduction); (c) Ipsilateral arm—sagittal plane (flexion); (d) Contralateral arm—frontal plane (abduction); (e) Contralateral arm—sagittal plane (flexion).

Progression 3: Single-Leg Stance with Ipsilateral/Contralateral Arm—Biceps Curl to Shoulder Press

This exercise is a variation of the progression 2 exercise. When designing and implementing strength-training programs, we need to have a bit of imagination to keep challenging the glutes. I could just keep adding pictures of various exercises, but that might defeat the object of what I am trying to demonstrate.

The patient stands on the dominant leg and lifts the other leg a few inches off the floor while holding a weight, as shown in figure 12.20(a). Once this position is maintained, the patient is instructed to flex the elbow of their ipsilateral arm (easier exercise) or their contralateral arm (harder exercise) to perform a biceps curl and to continue into a shoulder press, as shown in figures 12.20(b) and (c).

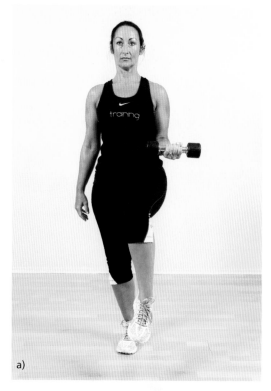

a)

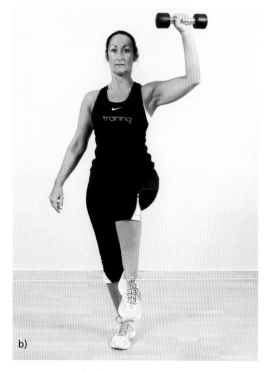

b)

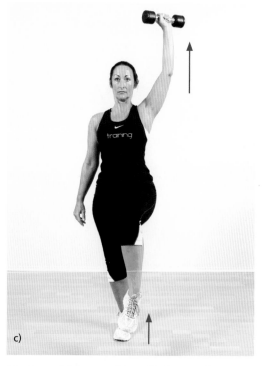

c)

Figure 12.20: Single-Leg Stance with Biceps Curl to Shoulder Press: (a) Start position; (b) Biceps curl; (c) Shoulder press.

Progression 4: Single-Leg Stance with Contralateral Cross-Over Arm Abduction

The patient stands on the dominant leg and lifts the other leg a few inches off the floor. They are asked to place their hand on the front of the hip of their dominant leg, as shown in figure 12.21(a). Once this position is maintained, the patient is instructed to lift their contralateral arm, starting from the dominant leg to cross over the body and finish in abduction (remaining in the frontal plane) for 10 reps, as shown in figure 12.21(b).

Knee bent.

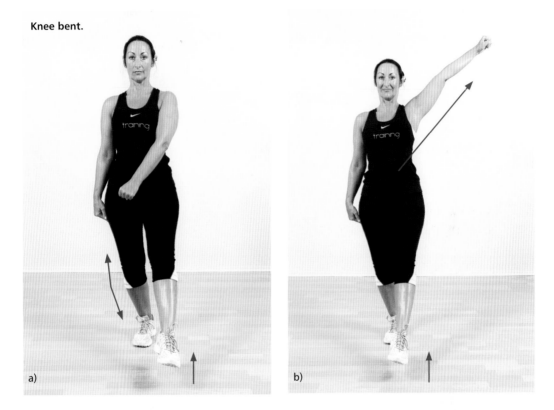

a)   b)

Figure 12.21: Single-Leg Stance with Contralateral Cross-Over Arm Abduction: (a) Start position; (b) Frontal plane (abduction).

Progression 5: Single-Leg Knee Bend with Contralateral Cross-Over Arm Abduction

The patient stands on the dominant leg and lifts the other leg a few inches off the floor (figure 2.17(a)). From this position of sustained balance, the patient bends the dominant knee to 30 degrees, as shown in figure 12.22(a). Once this position is maintained, the patient is instructed to lift their contralateral arm, starting from the dominant leg to cross over the body and finish in abduction, while they extend their knee to full extension at the same time, as shown in figure 12.22(b). The patient is asked to perform 10 reps.

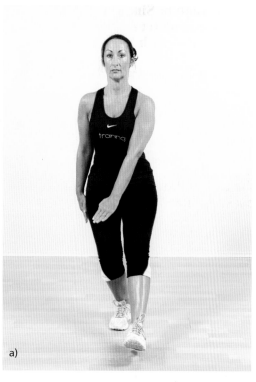

a)

Figure 12.22: Single-Leg Knee Bend with Contralateral Cross-Over Arm Abduction: (a) Start position; (b) Frontal plane (abduction); (c) With weight.

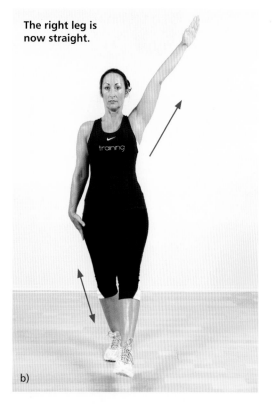

The right leg is now straight.

b)

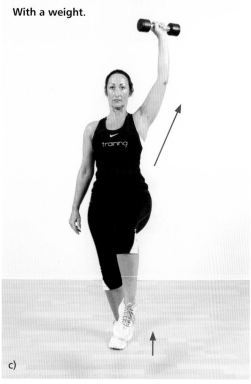

With a weight.

c)

Progression 6: Single-Leg Knee Bend with Contralateral Cross-Over Arm Abduction—with Weight

The patient performs the same exercise as in progression 5, but now holding a light weight (figure 12.22(c), page 174).

Core Ball Squat

A core ball is placed against the wall and the patient positions themselves so that the core ball is located near their lower back, as shown in figure 12.23(a). From this position, the patient steps forward slightly, with their knees shoulder-width apart. The patient is then asked to activate the inner core and slowly squat (eccentric phase) as shown in figure 12.23(b) until they reach a position of approximately 90 degrees, as shown in figure 12.23(c). The therapist makes sure that the tracking of the patella is toward the patient's second toe and that

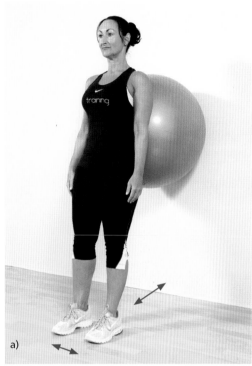

the patella does not pass beyond the level of the toes, as indicated by the arrows in figure 12.23(c). The patient is then instructed to stand up on the return (concentric phase) for a count of two. They are also instructed to squeeze their glutes just before the end phase of the squat.

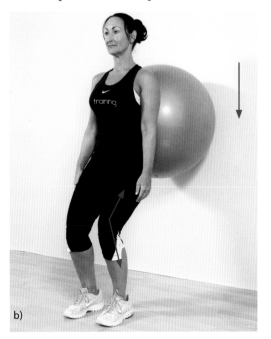

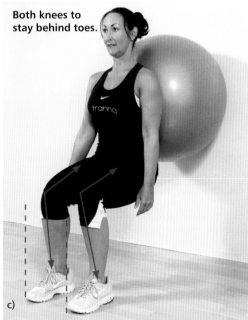

Both knees to stay behind toes.

Figure 12.23: Core Ball Squat: (a) Start position; (b) Half-squat position; (c) Full-squat position.

Progression 1: Core Ball Squat with Biceps Curl

The Core Ball Squat exercise is performed as explained above, except the patient now holds a light weight in each hand as shown in the start position in figure 12.24(a). During the concentric phase of the squat, the patient performs a biceps curl, as shown in figure 12.24(b). The finish position is shown in figure 12.24(c).

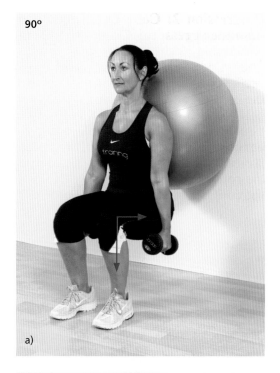

Figure 12.24: Core Ball Squat with Biceps Curl: (a) Start position; (b) Concentric phase of squat while curling the weight; (c) Finish position.

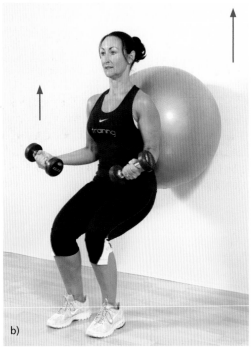

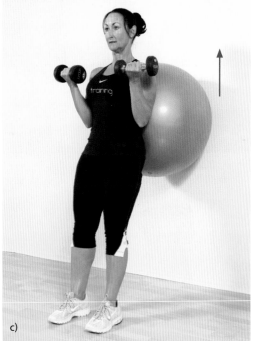

Progression 2: Core Ball Squat with Shoulder Press

The Core Ball Squat exercise is performed as explained above, except the patient now holds a light weight in each hand in a shoulder press position, as shown in figure 12.25(a). During the concentric phase of the squat, the patient performs a shoulder press, as shown in figure 12.25(b). The finish position is shown in figure 12.25(c).

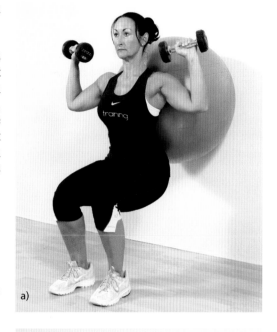
a)

Figure 12.25: Core Ball Squat with Shoulder Press: (a) Start position; (b) Concentric phase of squat while pressing the weight; (c) Finish position.

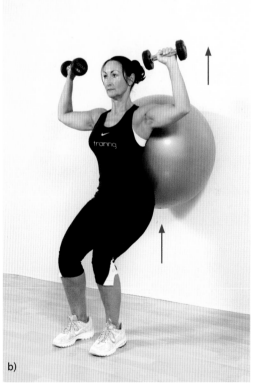
b)

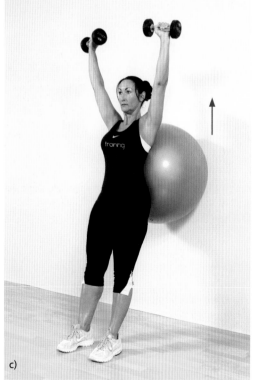
c)

Progression 3: Core Ball Isometric Squat with Forward Raise

The patient assumes the squat position shown in figure 12.23(c), holding a light weight in each hand. While maintaining this isometric (static) position, the patient is instructed to lift the right arm until it is parallel with the floor while the left arm is resting, as shown in figure 12.26(a). The right arm is then brought back to the start position, and the left arm lifted, as shown in figure 12.26(b). The whole process is repeated for the desired number of reps. There is no eccentric or concentric squatting motion during this exercise so the glutes are working isometrically to maintain the squat position.

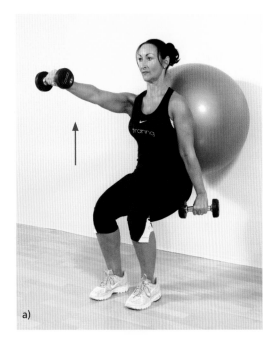 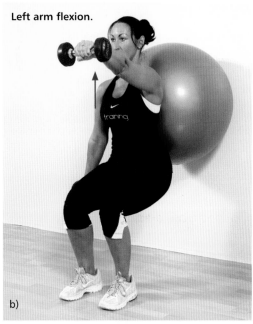

Figure 12.26: Core Ball Isometric Squat with Forward Raise: (a) Right arm is lifted; (b) Left arm is lifted.

Progression 4: Core Ball Squat with TheraBand

This progression is similar to the Core Ball Squat exercise, the only difference being that a TheraBand is placed around the outside of the patient's knee joints, as shown in figure 12.27(a). The patient is encouraged to abduct and externally rotate the hip joint into the TheraBand and hold this isometric position as they perform the squat, as shown in figures 12.27(b) and (c). Use of the TheraBand emphasizes the abduction and external rotation component of the Gmax and Gmed; there will also be a reciprocal inhibition of the adductors (switch of mechanism).

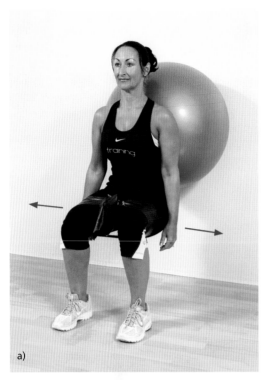

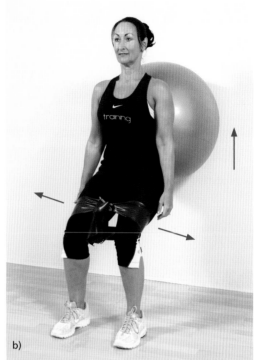

Figure 12.27: Core Ball Squat with TheraBand:
(a) Start position; (b) Midway position;
(c) Finish position.

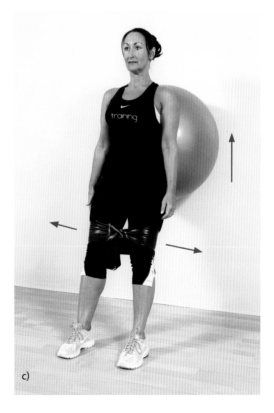

Progression 5: Core Ball Squat with TheraBand and Biceps Curl

This exercise is exactly the same as the squat with a core ball and a TheraBand placed around the patient's knees, except the patient now holds a light weight in each hand, as shown in figure 12.28(a). They are instructed to perform a squat from the 90-degree position to the finish position (concentric phase) while performing a biceps curl with the weight and applying resistance isometrically to the TheraBand, as shown in figure 12.28(b). The finish position is shown in figure 12.28(c).

Figure 12.28: Core Ball Squat with TheraBand and Biceps Curl: (a) Start position; (b) Concentric phase of squat while curling the weight; (c) Finish position.

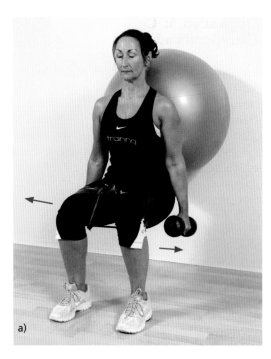

a)

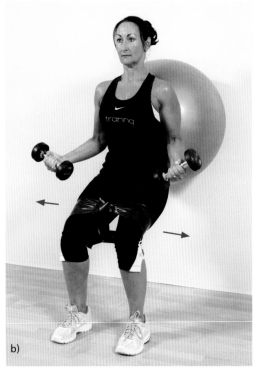

b)

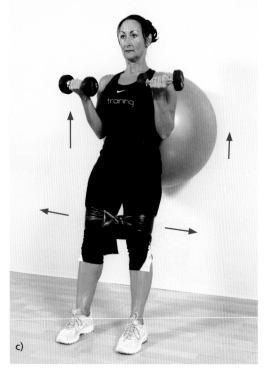

c)

Progression 6: Core Ball Squat with TheraBand and Shoulder Press

As a variation of progression 5, the patient holds a light weight in each hand in the shoulder press position, as shown in figure 12.29(a). The patient is then asked to perform a concentric squat movement from the 90-degree position while performing a shoulder press with the weight and applying resistance isometrically to the TheraBand, as shown in figure 12.29(b). The finish position is shown in figure 12.29(c).

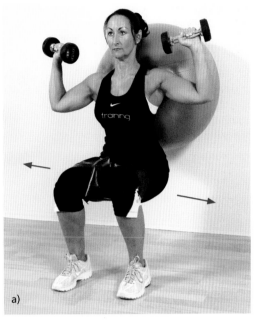

Figure 12.29: Core Ball Squat with TheraBand and Shoulder Press: (a) Start position; (b) Concentric phase of squat while pressing the weight; (c) Finish position.

a)

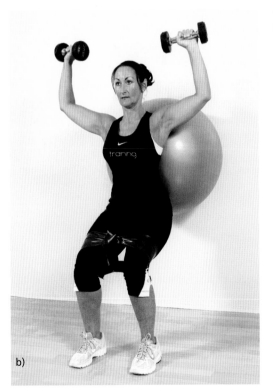

b)

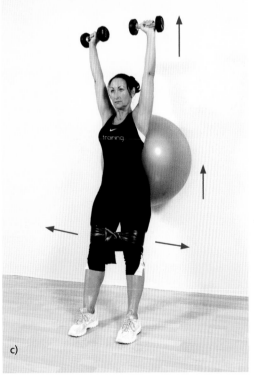

c)

Progression 7: Single-Leg Core Ball Squat

This progression is simply the Core Ball Squat exercise performed on one leg. A core ball is placed against the wall and the patient adopts a position so that the ball is located near their lower back as in the above exercises. From this position, the patient steps forward slightly, with their knees shoulder-width apart, and lifts their non-dominant leg a few inches off the floor, as shown in figure 12.30(a). They are instructed to slowly squat to 45 degrees, progressing to 90 degrees, as shown in figure 12.30(b).

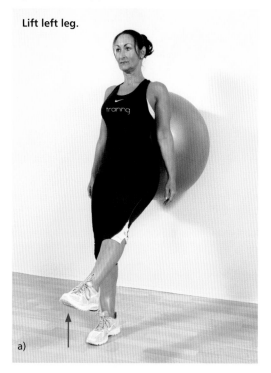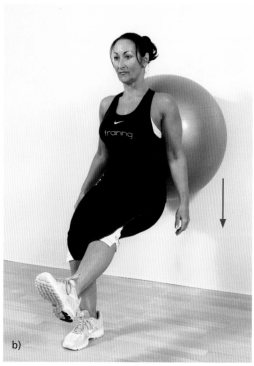

Figure 12.30: Single-Leg Core Ball Squat: (a) Start position; (b) 90-degree squat position.

Lateral Walk with TheraBand

The patient stands with their feet flat, their legs shoulder-width apart, and their back in a neutral position. A TheraBand is then placed around their mid-thigh, as shown in figure 12.31(a). The patient is asked to lift their non-dominant leg (so that they are balancing on the dominant leg) and to step to the side, as shown in figure 12.31(b). They are then instructed to return this leg to the start position, before repeating the same stepping movement with the other leg, as shown figure 12.31(c). Instead of the step to the side, a small lunge can be added later on.

Step left. **Step right.**

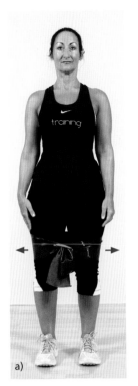
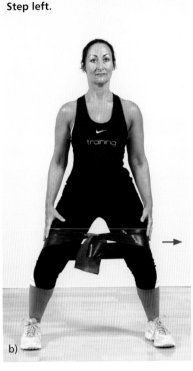
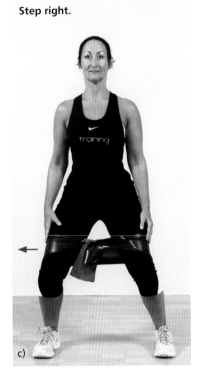

Figure 12.31: Lateral Walk with TheraBand:
(a) Start position; (b) Dominant leg fixed;
(c) Non-dominant leg fixed.

Single-Leg Squat

The patient stands with their feet flat, their legs shoulder-width apart, and their back facing a chair. They are asked to lift their non-dominant leg, so that they are balancing on the dominant leg. The patient is then instructed to slowly lower themselves down by performing a squat, as shown in figure 12.32. They continue to the point where their buttocks are in light contact with the chair, before slowly extending the hips to return to the start position.

Squat down.

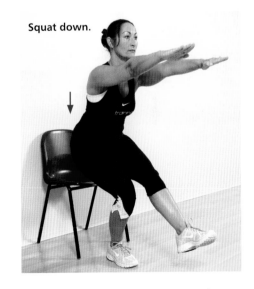

Figure 12.32: Single-Leg Squat into a Chair.

Step and Lunge Walk

This exercise combines the Gmax and Gmed—if I am honest, it is one of my favorite exercises.

Phase 1: Step

The patient stands with their legs shoulder-width apart, as shown in figure 12.33(a), and steps forward using the non-dominant leg, so that their foot is flat and in contact with the floor. The dominant leg is now positioned in such a way that the patient's balance is maintained by the toes of the dominant foot (figure 12.33(b)).

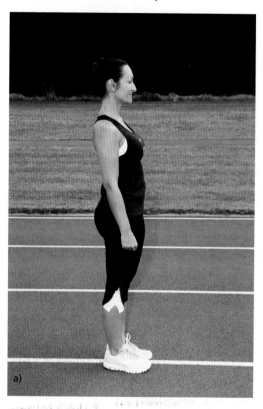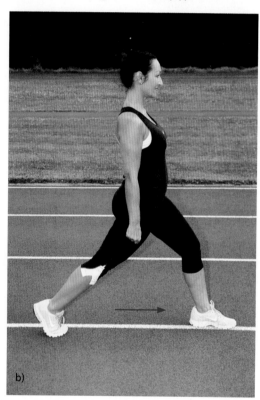

Figure 12.33: Step and Lunge Walk: (a): Phase 1—start position; (b) Phase 1—forward step.

Phase 2: Lunge

From the balanced position in figure 12.33(b), the patient is told to imagine that they are now holding in each hand a bucket of water which is full to the top. The patient is asked to lower the imaginary buckets to the floor without spilling any of the water. The therapist makes sure that the patient's knee does not pass the level of their toes and that it does not drift medially or laterally (figure 12.33(c)). If they are able, the patient repeats this lowering movement, before progressing to phase 3 of the exercise.

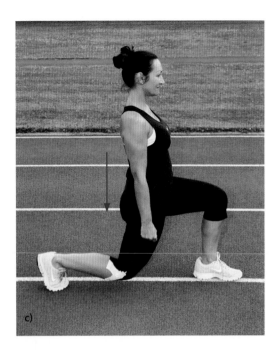

Figure 12.33: (c) Phase 2—lunge.

Phase 3: Hold

After the second repetition, the patient is instructed to rise from the lowered position (concentric phase) until the weight-bearing dominant leg is at full extension and the patient is in a state of controlled balance using the toes of the non-weight-bearing non-dominant leg (figure 12.33(d)).

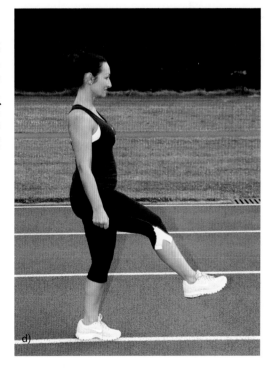

Figure 12.33: (d): Phase 3—hold.

Phase 4: Step to repeat

The step and lunge actions are now repeated with the opposite leg, as shown in figure 12.33(e).

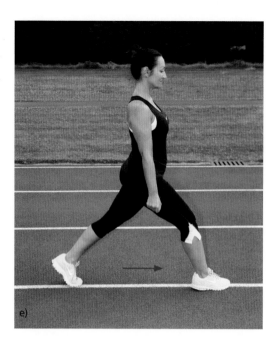

Figure 12.33: (e): Phase 4—step with opposite leg.

Progression 1: Thoracic Rotation

Once the patient has mastered the Step and Lunge Walk exercise, and they have good technique performing the specific movements, we can challenge the body by including some additional actions. This will start to activate and focus the brain on another exercise component and therefore take some of the emphasis away from the patient always having to consciously think about activating their glutes all the time while they exercise. The gluteal muscle group, once trained, should automatically contract as and when it is required to do so, rather than the conscious mind being forced to tell the glutes to switch on.

In this progression, the only difference to the Step and Lunge Walk exercise is that when the patient steps forward in phase 2, they are instructed to rotate their thoracic spine by using their arms, as shown in figure 12.34(a). When the patient moves on to perform phase 4, they rotate to the other side, as shown in figure 12.34(b).

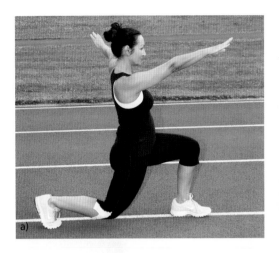
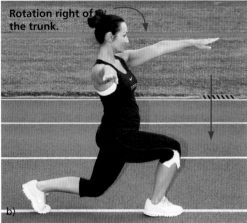

Figure 12.34: Step and Lunge Walk with Thoracic Rotation: (a) Rotation to the left; (b) Rotation to the right.

Progression 2: With Weight

In this progression of the Step and Lunge Walk exercise, the difference is the use of weights, for example dumbbells. The exercise is the same as before, but holding a weight in each hand: the patient steps forward and performs the lunge, with the dominant leg leading, as shown in figure 12.35(a). The exercise is then repeated using the non-dominant leg, as shown in figure 12.35(b).

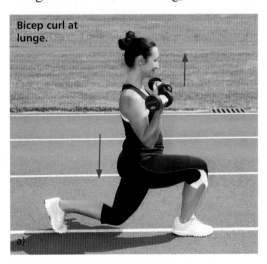
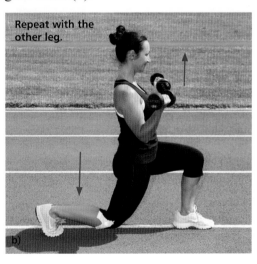

Figure 12.35: Step and Lunge Walk with Weights: (a) Dominant leg leading; (b) Non-dominant leg leading.

Double-Leg Bound

The patient stands on a line marked on the floor and slowly flexes at the hip into a squat position, as shown in figure 12.36(a). Keeping their spine in neutral, they are asked to bound or jump to the next marked line by extending at the hip, so that both feet are off the floor, as shown in figure 12.36(b). The therapist makes sure that when the patient lands on the second line, their knees are not allowed to drift medially or laterally, as this might indicate gluteal weakness. It must also be ensured that the patient's knees do not pass beyond the level of their toes, as shown in figure 12.36(c).

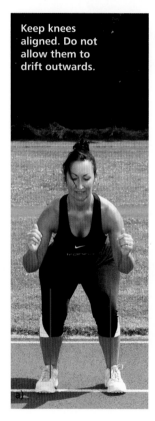
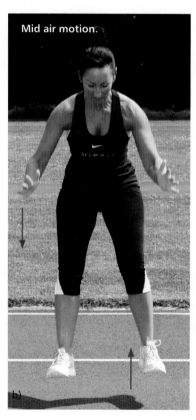
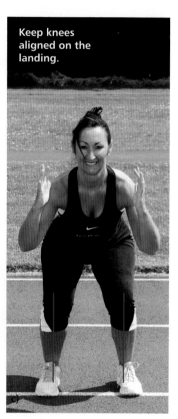

Figure 12.36: Double-Leg Bound: (a) Start position; (b) Mid-air position; (c) Finish position.

Single-Leg Dead Lift

The patient stands on their dominant leg and is asked to lift their non-dominant leg off the floor and into extension, as shown in figure 12.37(a). They are asked to slowly flex at the hip, keeping the back straight, in order to touch the floor with the opposite hand for a count of two, as shown in figure 12.37(b). The patient is then instructed to extend at the hip to the standing position for a count of two. The leg is kept straight, but it is permissible for it to be slightly bent in a case where hamstring tightness limits the ability to touch the floor.

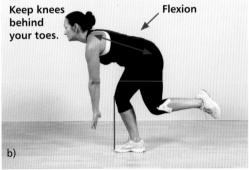

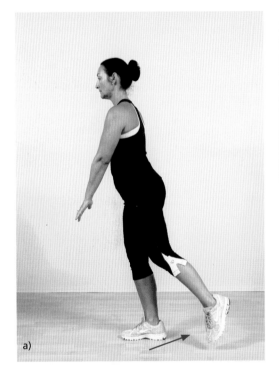

Figure 12.37: Single-Leg Dead Lift: (a) Start position; (b) Floor is touched with opposite hand.

Pelvic Drop

The patient stands on the edge of a 4" (10 cm) step with their dominant leg, as shown in figure 12.38(a). They are asked to dip their pelvis in order to lower the heel of the non-dominant leg, so that the foot touches the floor without bearing weight, as shown in figure 12.38(b). While keeping their hips and knees extended, the patient is instructed to return their foot to a position slightly higher than the height of the step, as shown in figure 12.38(c), in order to activate the Gmed.

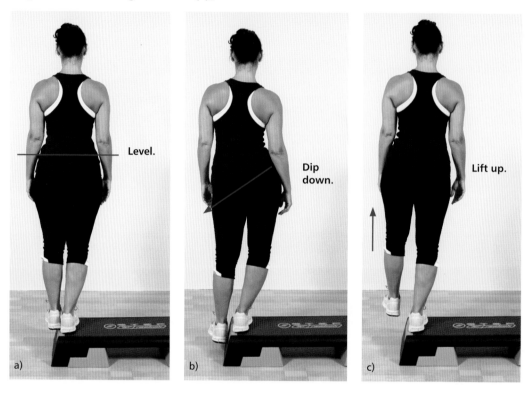

Figure 12.38: Pelvic Drop: (a) Start position; (b) Pelvis is dipped; (c) Finish position.

Forward Step-Up

The patient stands facing a 6–8" (15–20 cm) step, as shown in figure 12.39(a). They are instructed to step forward onto the step with their dominant leg leading (figure 12.39(b)) and then step forward and up with their non-dominant leg (figure 12.39(c)). The patient lowers their non-dominant leg back to the floor, followed by their dominant leg, and the process is repeated.

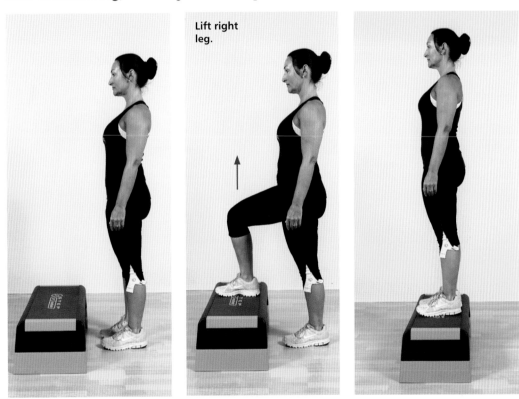

Figure 12.39: Forward Step-Up: (a) Start position; (b) Step with dominant leg; (c) Step with non-dominant leg.

Lateral Step-Down-Up

This exercise is similar to the forward step-up, but this time the patient stands sideways on top of a 6–8" (15–20 cm) step, as shown in figure 12.40(a). The patient is instructed to lift their dominant leg and put that foot on the floor (figure 12.40(b)). After contacting the floor, the leg is lifted and placed back on the step in the start position by the contraction of the glute of the non-dominant leg. The step movement is then repeated on the opposite side, as shown in figure 12.40(c).

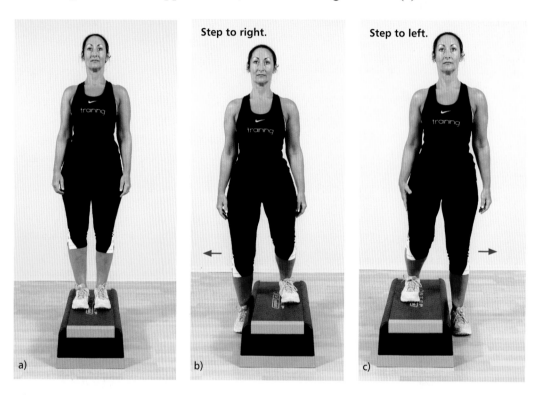

Figure 12.40: Lateral Step-Down-Up: (a) Start position; (b) Step with dominant leg; (c) Step with non-dominant leg.

Progression: Lateral Step-Down-Up with Lunge

This exercise is similar to the previous one, the only difference being that a lunge is now included. The patient is asked to lift their dominant leg and place that foot onto the floor. When the foot contacts the floor, the patient is instructed to perform a lunge (figure 12.41(a)). The leg is then lifted off the floor and placed back in the start position by the contraction of the glutes of the non-dominant leg. The step and lunge movement is then repeated on the opposite side, as shown in figure 12.41(b).

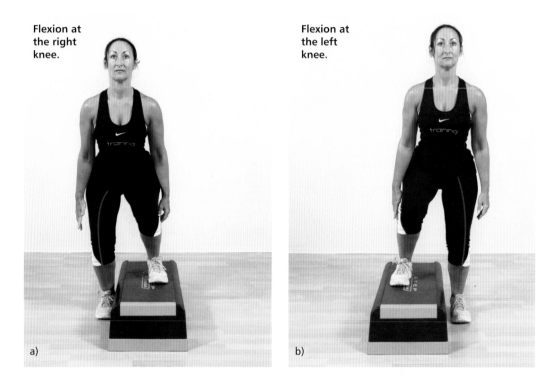

Figure 12.41: Lateral Step-Down-Up with Lunge: (a) Dominant leg; (b) Non-dominant leg.

Appendix: Gmax and Gmed Stabilization Exercise Sheet

The following exercises can be used in the physical therapist's own clinical setting. For each exercise there is a blank space in which a patient's repetitions and sets can be recorded.

Open Kinetic Chain

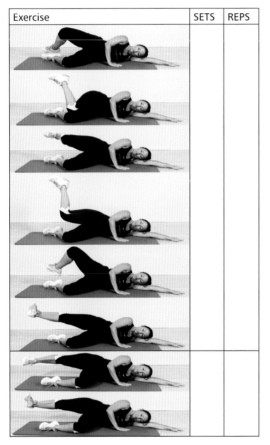

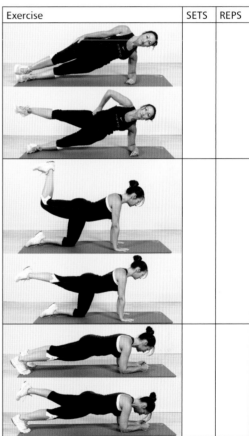

Closed Kinetic Chain

Exercise	SETS	REPS
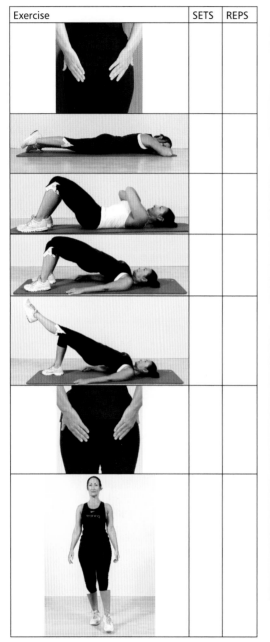		

Exercise	SETS	REPS
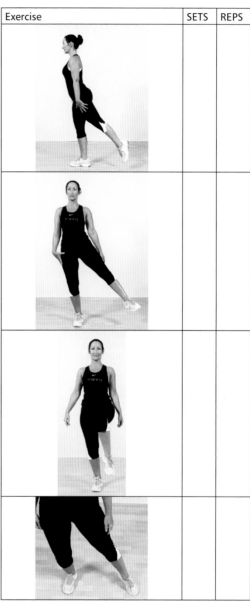		

Exercise	SETS	REPS
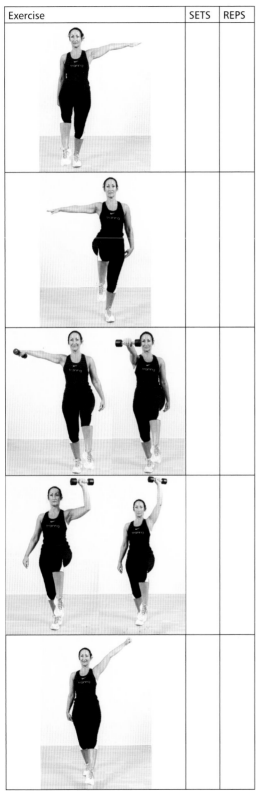		

Exercise	SETS	REPS
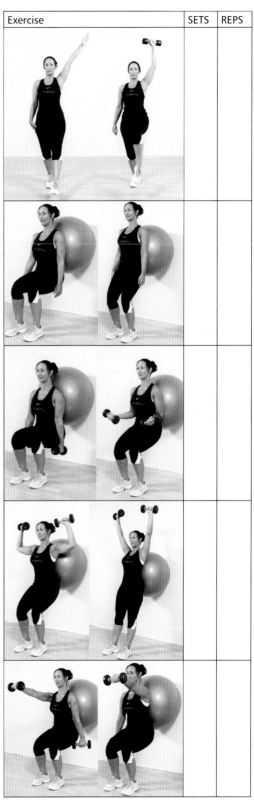		

Exercise	SETS	REPS

Exercise	SETS	REPS

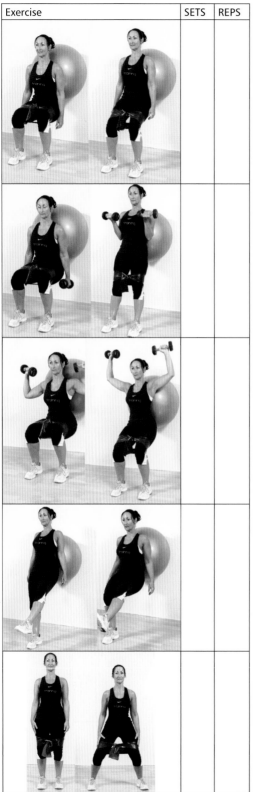

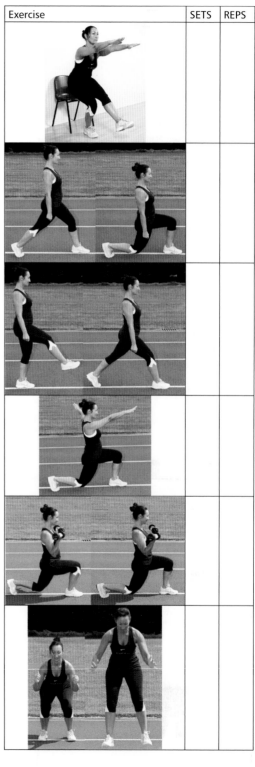

Exercise	SETS	REPS

Bibliography

Abernethy, B., Hanrahan, S., Kippers, V., et al. 2004. *The Biophysical Foundations of Human Movement*, Champaign, IL: Human Kinetics.

Ayotte, N., Stetts, D., Keenan, G., et al. 2007. "Electromyographical analysis of selected lower extremity muscles during 5 unilateral weight-bearing exercises," *J Orthop Sports Phys Ther* 37, 48–55.

Bauer, A.M., Webright, W.G., Arnold, B.L., et al. 1999. "Comparison of weight bearing and non-weight bearing gluteus medius EMG during an isometric hip abduction," *JAT* 34, S58.

Beckman, S.M., and Buchanan, T.S. 1995. "Ankle inversion injury and hyper mobility: Effect on hip and ankle muscle electromyography onset latency," *Arch Phys Med Rehab* 76, 1138–1143.

Bolgla, L., and Uhl, T. 2005. "Electromyographic analysis of hip rehabilitation exercises in a group of healthy subjects," *J Orthop Sports Phyl Ther* 35, 488–494.

Boren, K., Conrey, C., Le Coguic, J., et al. 2011. "Electromyographic analysis of gluteus medius and gluteus maximus during rehabilitation exercises," *Int J Sports Phys Ther* 6, 206–223.

Bullock-Saxton, J.E., Janda, V., and Bullock, M.I. 1994. "The influence of ankle sprain injury on muscle activation during hip extension," *Int J Sports Med* 15, 330–334.

Cailliet, R. 2003. *The Illustrated Guide to Functional Anatomy of the Musculoskeletal System*, Chicago, IL: American Medical Association.

Chaitow, L. 2006. *Muscle Energy Techniques*, 2nd edn, Edinburgh: Churchill Livingstone.

Chek, P. 2009. *An Integrated Approach to Stretching*, Vista, CA: C.H.E.K. Institute.

Dalton, E. 2014. Short leg syndrome, part 1, Author website.

Distefano, L., Blackburn, J., Marshall, S., et al. 2009. "Gluteal activation during common therapeutic exercises," *J Orthop Sports Phys Ther* 39, 532–540.

Earl, J.E. 2005. "Gluteus medius activity during three variations of isometric single-leg stance," *J Sport Rehabil* 14, 1–11.

Earls, J., and Myers, T. 2010. *Fascial Release for Structural Balance*, Chichester, UK/Berkeley, CA: Lotus Publishing/North Atlantic Books.

Elphinston, J. 2013. *Stability, Sport and Performance Movement*, Chichester, UK/Berkeley, CA: Lotus Publishing/North Atlantic Books.

Fredericson, M., Cookingham, C.L., Chaudhari, A.M., et al. 2000. "Hip abductor weakness in distance runners with iliotibial band syndrome," *Clin J Sport Med* 10, 169–175.

Friel, K., McLean, N., Myers, C., and Caceras, M. 2006. "Ipsilateral hip abductor weakness after inversion ankle sprain," *J Athl Train* 41, 74–78.

Fryette, H.H. 1918. "Physiological movements of the spine," *J Am Osteopath Assoc* 18, 1–2.

Garrick, J.G. 1977. "The frequency of injury, mechanism of injury, and epidemiology of ankle sprains," *Am J Sports Med* 5, 241–242.

Gibbons, J. 2008. "Preparing for glory," *International Therapist* 81, 14–16.

Gibbons, J. 2009. "Putting maximus back into the gluteus," *International Therapist* 87, 32–33.

Gibbons, J. 2011. *Muscle Energy Techniques: A Practical Guide for Physical Therapists*, Chichester, UK: Lotus Publishing.

Hammer, W.I. 1999. *Functional Soft Tissue Examination and Treatment by Manual Methods: New Perspectives*, 2nd edn, Gaithersburg, MD: Aspen.

Hertel, J., Sloss, B.R., and Earl, J.E. 2005. "Effect of foot orthotics on quadriceps and gluteus medius electromyographic activity during selected exercises," *Arch Phys Med Rehab* 86, 26–30.

Hungerford, B., Gilleard, W., and Hodges, P. 2003. "Evidence of altered muscle recruitment in the presence of posterior pelvic pain and failed load transfer through the pelvis," *Spine* 28, 1593–1600.

Ireland, M.L., Wilson, J.D., Ballantyne, B.T., and Davis, I.M. 2003. "Hip strength in females with and without patellofemoral pain," *J Orthop Sports Phys Ther* 33, 671–676.

Janda, V. 1983. *Muscle Function Testing.* London: Butterworth-Heinemann.

Janda, V. 1987. "Muscles and motor control in low back pain: Assessment and management," in Twomey, L.T. (ed.), *Physical Therapy of the Low Back*, New York: Churchill Livingstone, 253–278.

Janda, V. 1992. "Treatment of chronic low back pain," *J Man Med* 6, 166–168.

Janda, V. 1996. "Evaluation of muscular imbalance," in Liebenson, C. (ed.), *Rehabilitation of the Spine: A Practitioner's Manual*, 1st edn, Baltimore, MD: Lippincott, Williams & Wilkins, 97–112.

Jarmey, C. 2006. *The Concise Book of the Moving Body*, Chichester, UK/Berkeley, CA: Lotus Publishing/North Atlantic Books.

Jarmey, C. 2008. *The Concise Book of Muscles*, 2nd edn, Chichester, UK/Berkeley, CA: Lotus Publishing/North Atlantic Books.

Kankaanpaa, M., Taimela, S., Laaksonen, D., et al. 1998. "Back and hip extensor fatigability in chronic low back pain patients and controls," *Archives Phys Med Rehab* 79, 412–417.

Kendall, F.P., McCreary, E.K., Provance, P.G., et al. 2010. *Muscle Testing and Function with Posture and Pain*, 5th edn, Baltimore, MD: Lippincott, Williams & Wilkins.

Leavey, V.J., Sandrey, M.A., and Dahmer, G. 2010. "Comparative effects of 6-week balance, gluteus medius strength, and combined programs on dynamic postural control," *J Sport Rehabil* 19, 268–287.

Lee, D.G. 2004. *The Pelvic Girdle: An Approach to the Examination and Treatment of the Lumbopelvic-Hip Region*, Edinburgh: Churchill Livingstone.

Lehman, G.J., Lennon, D., Tresidder, B., et al. 2004. "Muscle recruitment patterns during the prone leg extension," *BMC Musculoskel Disord* 5, 3.

Maitland, J. 2001. *Spinal Manipulation Made Simple: A Manual of Soft Tissue Techniques*, Berkeley, CA: North Atlantic Books.

Martin, C. 2002. *Functional Movement Development*, 2nd edn, London: W.B. Saunders Co.

Mitchell, F.L., Sr. 1948. "The balanced pelvis and its relationship to reflexes," *Academy of Applied Osteopathy Year Book 1948*, pp. 146–151.

Norris, C.M. 2011. *Managing Sports Injuries: A Guide for Students and Clinicians*, 4th edn, Edinburgh and New York: Churchill Livingstone.

Ogiwara, S., and Sugiura, K. 2001. "Determination of ten-repetition-maximum for gluteus medius muscle," *J Phys Ther Sci* 13, 53–57.

Osar, E. 2012. *Corrective Exercise Solutions to Common Hip and Shoulder Dysfunction*, Chichester, UK: Lotus Publishing.

O'Sullivan, K., Smith, S.M., and Sainsbury, D. 2010. "Electromyographic analysis of the three subdivisions of gluteus medius during weight-bearing exercises," *Sports Med, Arthroscopy, Rehab, Ther & Technol* 2, 17.

O'Sullivan, P., Twomey, L., Allison, G., et al. 1997. "Altered pattern of abdominal muscle activation in patients with chronic low back pain," *Austral J Physiother* 43(2), 91–98.

Pierce, N., and Lee, W.A. 1990. "Muscle firing order during active prone hip extension," *J Orthop Sports Phys Ther* 12, 2–9.

Richardson, C., Jull, G., Hodges, P., and Hides, J. 1999. *Therapeutic Exercise for Spinal Segmental Stabilization in Low Back Pain: Scientific Basis and Clinical Approach*, Edinburgh: Churchill Livingstone.

Sahrman, S. 2002. *Diagnosis and Treatment of Movement Impairment Syndromes*, 1st edn, St. Louis, MO: Mosby Inc.

Schmitz, R.J., Riemann, B.L., and Thompson, T. 2002. "Gluteus medius activity during isometric closed-chain hip rotation," *J Sport Rehabil* 11, 179–188.

Sherrington, C.S. 1907. "On reciprocal innervation of antagonistic muscles," *Proc R Soc Lond [Biol]* 79B, 337.

Smith, R.W., and Reischl, S.F. 1986. "Treatment of ankle sprains in young athletes," *Am J Sports Med* 14, 465–471.

Thomas, C.L. 1997. *Taber's Cyclopaedic Medical Dictionary*, 18th edn, Philadelphia, PA: F.A. Davis.

Umphred, D.A., Byl, N., Lazaro, R.T., and Roller, M. 2001. "Interventions for neurological disabilities," in Umphred, D.A. (ed.), *Neurological Rehabilitation*, 4th edn, St. Louis, MO: Mosby Inc., 56–134.

Wilmore, J.H., and Costill, D.L. 1994. *Physiology of Sport & Exercise*, Champaign, IL: Human Kinetics.

Wolfe, M.W., Uhl, T.L., Mattacola, C.G., and McCluskey, L.C. 2001. "Management of ankle sprains," *Am Fam Physician* 63, 93–104.

Index